The Neuropsychology Toolkit

Richard L. Wanlass

The Neuropsychology Toolkit

Guidelines, Formats, and Language

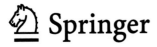 Springer

Richard L. Wanlass
University of California, Davis, Medical Center
Sacramento, CA, USA
Richard.Wanlass@ucdmc.ucdavis.edu

ISBN 978-1-4614-1881-8   e-ISBN 978-1-4614-1882-5
DOI 10.1007/978-1-4614-1882-5
Springer New York Dordrecht Heidelberg London

Library of Congress Control Number: 2011944429

Printed on acid-free paper

Springer is part of Springer Science+Business Media (www.springer.com)

Introduction

Neuropsychology is not a particularly forgiving profession. The stakes of our evaluations are often high. Costly damage claims or disability awards may hinge on our findings. Our reports can form the basis on which rights and autonomy are denied for some, or the basis on which legal responsibility is absolved for others. Some patients and family members take offense when we identify cognitive impairment, and some take exception when we do not. Carefully built reputations may come under attack when attorneys hire neuropsychology experts to scrutinize our scoring, critique our test selection, and contradict our interpretations. And the paper trail of our work is always long, not only the records we must retain, but also the transcripts of our depositions and court testimony, which seemingly survive into perpetuity.

All of which makes for a challenging and meaningful profession, but one in which minimizing mistakes is generally preferable to learning from them the hard way. This manual is offered with the intention of helping new and developing neuropsychology practitioners minimize errors, omissions, and misconceptions and move more rapidly and painlessly towards proficiency.

Part I presents guidelines for improving the assessment and reporting process, with the rationale for each guideline, correct and incorrect examples, and exceptions or clarifications as needed.

Part II provides tools for gathering background information and writing reports more efficiently and clearly.

And Part III proposes wording for use in difficult-to-write sections of neuropsychological reports.

Acknowledgments

My thanks to the 100 or so neuropsychology interns, fellows, and staff I have had the pleasure of supervising and training. It is their motivation to learn and improve that inspired my efforts to develop and refine the tools in this manual. A few deserve special recognition for their contributions to this process:

Robin Timm, Ph.D.
Erik Lande, Ph.D.
Elizabeth Houghton-Faryna, Psy.D.
David Broome, Psy.D.
Renee Low, Ph.D.
Ashley Gunter, Psy.D.
Brandon Adams, Psy.D.
Sharon Perlman, Psy.D.
June Paltzer, Ph.D.
Louisa Parks, Psy.D.
Jane McClay, Psy.D.
Brenda Havellana, Psy.D.

Inasmuch as they may prefer anonymity, the many supervisees who inspired the how-not-to examples herein are acknowledged collectively.

Special thanks to Susan Wanlass, Ph.D., Professor of English at California State University, Sacramento, for expert consultation in the area of writing style.

And last but certainly not least, thanks to the neuropsychologists whose excellent instruction first inspired me:

Robert Deysach, Ph.D.
William Lynch, Ph.D.
James Moses, Ph.D.

Feedback: This handbook will undoubtedly elicit reader comments regarding my own errors, omissions, and misconceptions, and I invite submission of these to NeuRules@gmail.com.

About the Author

Currently I serve as Chief Psychologist and Clinical Professor in the Department of Physical Medicine and Rehabilitation at the University of California, Davis, Medical Center. Prior to arriving here in 1987, I directed neuropsychological and psychological services in a CARF-accredited free-standing brain injury rehabilitation center. Other previous activities include 15 years of part-time private practice, consultation to brain injury rehabilitation programs, and service as an Expert Reviewer for the California Board of Psychology. I am honored to have been elected a Fellow of the National Academy of Neuropsychology.

Contents

Part I
NeuRules: Guidelines for Improving Assessment and Reporting

In the course of training and supervising interns, postdoctoral fellows, and neuro-psychologists over the past quarter century, I have noted many recurring errors, omissions, and misconceptions that diminish the quality of neuropsychological evaluations. The following guidelines, or "NeuRules," are offered to help readers identify, understand, and avoid some of these problems.

This collection is by no means exhaustive, and readers are encouraged to develop their own supplemental guidelines as they achieve further insights into ways to improve their work. Suggestions for additional NeuRules to be included in future editions of this manual are welcome and can be sent to NeuRules@gmail.com.

Please note that these guidelines are intended to supplement rather than replace existing laws and professional ethics and standards. In cases in which there is a conflict between the guidance offered herein and applicable laws, ethics, or standards, the reader is advised to assign precedence to legal requirements and professional ethics and standards.

Also, as those who have witnessed lively interchanges on neuropsychology listservs are aware, this is a field with some fairly strong divergences of opinion about the proper way to practice. Therefore, readers should recognize that some supervisors may have different perspectives on a few of these guidelines.

Chapter 1
Pre-Test

Before reading these guidelines, you are encouraged to take a half-hour to complete the pre-test presented on the following pages. Then, when you have finished reviewing the guidelines portion of the manual, you will have a chance to take a post-test to demonstrate what you have learned.

R.L. Wanlass, *The Neuropsychology Toolkit: Guidelines, Formats, and Language*,
DOI 10.1007/ 978-1-4614-1882-5_1, © Springer Science+Business Media, LLC 2012

Glasscow Comma Scale Pre-Test

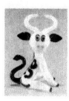

This brief report contains more than 60 errors reflecting limitations in psychological and medical <u>knowledge</u>, <u>writing ability</u>, and <u>common sense</u>. Please correct as many errors (including errors of both <u>commission</u> and <u>omission</u>) as you can in the next 30 minutes and then list your name and the date on the line at the bottom of the last page. Please switch to a pen or pencil that writes in a different color after 15 minutes.

Wudzit Taique, a 47 year old Latvian woman recently provisionally

diagnosed with Dementia of the Alzheimer's Type (DAT) was referred by

Dr. Edward S. Hands, M.D. for this 01/01/2011 neuropychological evaluation.

Prior to her symptom onset, Ms. Taique reported being extremely active (i.e.

liked to paint, make stained glass, and attending the opera) but she tearfully

related that she is no longer interested in these hobbies. Her recent activities have consisted only of sipping vodka and watching Fox News.

Her husband, a long-haul tractor-trailer driver and stamp collector, reports

observing cognitive symptoms in his wife for the past six months. He also said

she will emit gasping and snorting sounds when she sleeps.

They live locally with there preschool-age grandchild, who they adopted

following the death of the child's parents last year.

Ms. Taique immigrated from Latvia two years ago. She completed 12 years

of schooling in Russian and Mining Technology. She then worked as a coal minor

for several years until developing chronic back pain from a 1975 mining accident.

Currently prescribed medications consist of Oxycontin, Nardil, and

Hydrocodone, and she discontinued Luvox two days ago due to side affects.

She also takes about two asprin every four to six hours.

Ms. Taique's vision was determined to be adequate to participate in testing, as was her hearing, despite her complaint of tinnitis. Test results are considered

a valid reflection of her current cognitive ability.

Her Full Scale IQ is 112 (VCI = 107; PRI = 103; WMI = 104; PSI = 105).

Thus, Ms. Taique's current overall intellectual functioning tested as superior, with

verbal abilities significantly stronger than nonverbal abilities. She demonstrated

relative strength in arithmetic, as indicated by her Digit Span scaled score of 12,

which falls at the 84th%ile. On the Trail Making Test, Mr. Taique scored in the

mild-deficit range (32nd%ile) compared to others her age group, however, this

measure is not particularly sensitive to neurologic dysfunction. Language abilities

appeared intact, as performance on multiple measures of reading, spelling, comprehension, design fluency, and word-finding abilities were normal. Memory

testing revealed deficits in list learning and free recall, while recognition tested as normal, suggesting problems involving both retention and retrieval.

Ms. Taique scored in the normal range (T=67) on Scale 7 of the MMPI-2,

and there are no other indications of depression.

In conclusion, assessment results are consistent with a diagnosis of DAT.

Chapter 2
Interacting with Others

A Referral Sources

Rule I-A01: Make sure you know who the real referral source is, as sometimes a primary care physician is required by an insurance company to formally make the referral, whereas the professional actually wanting to see the results is a specialist such as a psychiatrist, physiatrist, or neurologist.

> *Rationale*: Appropriate patient care may be delayed if your report is not received by the professional who initiated the request for the evaluation.

> *Exceptions or Clarifications*: Often it is appropriate to also provide a copy of the report to the primary care physician, even when a specialist initiated the referral.

Rule I-A02: When accepting referrals from attorneys, be especially careful to establish who is responsible for payment.

> *Rationale*: You are more likely to be paid and to avoid accusations of inappropriate billing.

> *Incorrect Example*: Accepting a referral from an attorney for a forensic evaluation and billing the insurance company without establishing with the insurance company that the service will be covered.

> *Correct Example*: Clarifying with the attorney and patient who will be responsible for the bill and, if appropriate, obtaining payment or a retainer in advance.

Rule I-A03: Ascertain the manner in which your referral source wishes to receive results.

> *Rationale*: Patient care is likely to be enhanced if results are delivered in the manner most convenient for the referral source.

R.L. Wanlass, *The Neuropsychology Toolkit: Guidelines, Formats, and Language,*
DOI 10.1007/ 978-1-4614-1882-5_2, © Springer Science+Business Media, LLC 2012

Exceptions or Clarifications: Some referral sources wish to have the test results faxed for more rapid delivery, while others prefer to have the results mailed in order to have a more legible report and in order not to overload their fax machines. If a report is faxed, find out if the referral source also wants a copy to be mailed.

Do not fax without first carefully verifying the accuracy of the fax number, and then double-check the number you have entered before pushing the "send" button on the fax machine. Comply with any applicable policies or regulations regarding the electronic transmission of confidential patient information.

Some referral sources may, in certain cases, prefer to receive telephone feedback, possibly even before the report is completed. Some may also have preferences about the length of the report that they find most helpful.

Rule I-A04: List appropriate titles and/or degrees of your referral sources in reports.

Rationale: People who pursue advanced degrees in fields such as healthcare generally appreciate having their credentials listed and may be more likely to keep referring if shown this courtesy.

Incorrect Example: Referring to a doctorate holder as "Mr. Smith" or "John Smith."

Correct Example: "Dr. Smith" or "John Smith, M.D."

Exceptions or Clarifications: Do not list both title and degree unless submitting your report to a professional who has demonstrated a preference for such redundancy in his or her own communications (e.g., Dr. John Smith, D.C.).

B   Support Staff

Rule I-B01: When operating within an institution, be especially courteous towards and respectful of support staff involved in scheduling patients, checking patients in, transcribing reports, and billing.

Rationale: In addition to contributing to a more enjoyable working environment, courtesy and respect for support staff may increase their motivation to be helpful towards you and your patients.

Rule I-B02: Be courteous towards support staff working in other offices (e.g., colleagues, referral sources).

Rationale: Courtesy towards support staff in other offices may increase their motivation to assist in transmitting information between you and the other professional (e.g., providing records), obtaining authorizations or payments, and directing future referrals to you.

C   Patients

Rule I-C01: Recognize that patients referred for neuropsychological evaluation may have cognitive deficits and/or resource limitations that make it difficult for them to keep scheduled appointments, and make appropriate accommodations for this.

> *Rationale*: You will be less likely to experience no-shows.
>
> *Incorrect Example*: Scheduling an appointment by telephone with a patient being referred for memory impairment and trusting that the patient will arrive.
>
> *Correct Example*: Arranging the appointment, if necessary, with a family member and following up with written and/or telephone confirmation and reminders.
>
> *Exceptions or Clarifications*: Observe appropriate confidentiality practices when contacting parties other than the patient.

Rule I-C02: Make sure that you verify and document that the patient or guardian understands the purpose and nature of the evaluation, potential uses of the results, and limitations in confidentiality.

> *Rationale*: Professional ethics and legal statutes generally mandate adherence to this rule. In addition, cooperation with the evaluation may be improved if the patient understands the purpose of testing.
>
> *Exceptions or Clarifications*: Some patients may be too cognitively limited to fully appreciate these issues, and in such cases it is advisable to also provide explanation and obtain consent from a responsible family member even when no formal guardianship has been established by the court.
>
> When guardianship or conservatorship is claimed, verify this through examination of the relevant legal document and document that you have done so.
>
> When evaluating a child of divorced parents, verify which parent has legal authority to give consent for the evaluation and who has a right to receive disclosure of results.
>
> When the evaluation is being conducted at the request of a third party such as a judge, hearing officer, or disability insurance company, clarify to the examinee who the actual "client" is and who will be entitled to receive the evaluation findings and report.

D   Family Members

Rule I-D01: When possible be inclusive of and courteous towards family members.

> *Rationale*: Cooperation of family members is frequently useful for gathering background information, ensuring that the patient comes to scheduled appointments, and implementing recommendations.

Exceptions or Clarifications: Follow applicable legal and ethical guidelines, including obtaining consent from the patient to communicate with family. In cases in which a family member asserts a right to receive information, but the patient does not consent, verify the family member's legal authority (e.g., conservatorship documentation).

E   Payers

Rule I-E01: Verify insurance coverage or other payment agreements, or else make sure support personnel have done so.

Rationale: Insurance companies differ widely in terms of what services/CPT codes they reimburse, the number of billable hours they consider appropriate for a neuropsychological evaluation, whether pre-authorization is required, and the amount they pay.

Exceptions or Clarifications: Even in self-pay cases, clear delineation of services and costs, preferably with written documentation of the agreement, can prevent misunderstandings and complaints.

Chapter 3
Managing Environmental Considerations

Rule II-01: Maintain a quiet and comfortable testing environment as free as possible from distractions.

Rationale: Normative data are usually gathered under such conditions, and your test results will be more meaningful if gathered in a similar manner.

Incorrect Example: Leaving a telephone ringer on, failing to put up a do-not-disturb sign on the door, or allowing the testing room to be too hot or too cold.

Exceptions or Clarifications: There may be occasions in which observation of an examinee in a noisy or otherwise distracting environment, such as a cafeteria, provides useful data, although appropriate caution will be needed in interpreting such observational data in the absence of formal norms.

Rule II-02: Maintain a neat and orderly testing environment.

Rationale: A neat and orderly testing environment will help to convey an image of professionalism, which may result in better compliance by the examinee with the testing process. Such an environment may also result in more favorable comments about the testing experience by the examinee to the referral source, which may increase the likelihood of future referrals. An uncluttered environment is also likely to be less distracting to the examinee.

Incorrect Example: Leaving food or other nonprofessional personal items in view.

Correct Example: Keeping work surfaces relatively free of clutter.

Rule II-03: Keep records of other patients or any other items containing patient names in a secure location where your examinee will not see them.

Rationale: Not doing so violates ethical standards regarding patient confidentiality and also undermines your examinee's trust that you will keep his or her records confidential.

Incorrect Example: Leaving other patient files on a desk in the exam room or showing your examinee a page in your appointment calendar that lists names of other patients.

Correct Example: Protecting patient identity and clinical data from other patients.

R.L. Wanlass, *The Neuropsychology Toolkit: Guidelines, Formats, and Language*,
DOI 10.1007/ 978-1-4614-1882-5_3, © Springer Science+Business Media, LLC 2012

Rule II-04: Keep test manuals and other test materials secure so that examinees do not examine or take information that the test developer intended to be viewed only by professionals.

> *Rationale*: Failure to adequately safeguard test security is a violation of ethical standards, and often a violation of the agreement made with the test publisher when the materials were purchased. If test security is not maintained, and an examinee has already seen test content, the results of testing may be less valid.

Rule II-05: Do not leave examinees alone in the exam room unless you have made certain that all confidential patient information and protected test materials are secure.

> *Rationale*: Protection of confidential patient information and test security.

Rule II-06: Maintain a safe testing environment.

> *Rationale*: Removing environmental hazards will decrease the likelihood of harm to either your examinee or you.

> *Incorrect Example*: Leaving extension cords or other items where you or the examinee might trip on them or not securing overhead items that might fall.

> *Correct Example*: Removing scissors or other potential weapons that a frustrated examinee might use against you and making sure that the examinee's chair is not on rollers or otherwise unstable.

Rule II-07: A well-lit testing environment is important, especially for older subjects, but attempt to find a balance between illumination and glare, and also be mindful of some examinees' photophobia.

> *Rationale*: To increase the validity of test results.

Chapter 4
Obtaining and Reporting Background Information

A Identifying Information

Rule III-A01: In hospital settings or other settings subject to Joint Commission standards, verify your examinee's identity. Also do so in any circumstance in which an examinee might have an incentive to send another person for testing in his or her place.

> *Rationale*: Verification of patient identification is a standard enforced by the Joint Commission. In an effort to obtain benefits or services, or evade responsibility or consequences, an examinee could subvert the evaluation process by sending someone else to be tested in his or her stead.

> *Exceptions or Clarifications*: Simple methods of the verifying a patient's identity include examination of a driver's license or other picture identification or examination of a patient ID wristband (in inpatient settings).

Rule III-A02: Calculate the examinee's actual age based on his or her date of birth and the current date, rather than relying solely on self-report, family report, or another medical provider's statement of age.

> *Rationale*: Patients, family members, and other medical providers may be inaccurate, and it is preferable not to perpetuate inaccuracy, especially when doing so may lead to selection of an inappropriate normative comparison group.

> *Exceptions or Clarifications*: When discrepancies are noted, double-check your own calculations and attempt to find corroboration that you have identified the correct date of birth. In rare cases in which conclusive determination of actual date of birth is not possible, note this in your report and take this uncertainty into account in reaching conclusions about test results.

R.L. Wanlass, *The Neuropsychology Toolkit: Guidelines, Formats, and Language*,
DOI 10.1007/ 978-1-4614-1882-5_4, © Springer Science+Business Media, LLC 2012

B   Reason for Referral

Rule III-B01: If you are unsure of the reason for referral, contact the referral source for clarification.

> *Rationale*: The value of your reports will be judged in large measure upon the degree to which you have answered the questions of concern to the referring party, even when those questions have not been well delineated for you.

> *Exceptions or Clarifications*: Alternatively, sometimes the reason for referral can be discerned through review of recent records.

C   History of Presenting Problem

Rule III-C01: In traumatic brain injury cases, carefully document self-report and medical evidence regarding alteration in consciousness at the time of the injury.

> *Rationale*: This information can be useful in establishing the severity of the injury and is of particular importance in cases of alleged mild traumatic brain injury.

> *Incorrect Example*: Ms. Lopez sustained a loss of consciousness.

> *Correct Example*: Ms. Lopez reported a loss of consciousness for an estimated 30 seconds, and this self-report is consistent with evidence in the paramedic's report. Ms. Lopez reported being confused and dazed at the scene of the accident, with only a vague memory of the events that transpired until she arrived in the emergency room. She said her memory is fairly continuous for the events that happened thereafter.

> *Exceptions or Clarifications*: Be careful to check for available sources of information besides patient report, and utilize appropriate skepticism when dealing with cases in which the patient has a financial incentive to magnify the severity of the injury. Try to distinguish between what the patient truly recalls and what he or she may have heard from others or what he or she believes must have happened.

> Attempt to gather information about alteration in consciousness and subsequent cognitive difficulties associated with prior injuries as well.

Rule III-C02: When reporting a list of problems, phrase each item of the list in a consistent manner so that you do not intermix abilities with deficiencies.

> *Rationale*: To facilitate reader understanding.

> *Incorrect Examples*: She reported difficulty with finding words, remembering names of acquaintances, and using "nonsense words."

> Medical records indicate that Mr. Hassan has trouble with balance, gait, and overall weakness.

> *Correct Examples*: She reported difficulty with finding words and remembering names of acquaintances. She also reported that she sometimes uses "nonsense words."

Medical records indicate that Mr. Hassan has trouble with balance, gait, and overall strength.

Rule III-C03: Be alert to the distinction commonly made in medical settings between "signs," which are more observable and objective, and "symptoms," which are more subjective and experiential.

Rationale: To communicate more effectively with professional colleagues.

Incorrect Example: Symptoms of depression observed during the interview include tearfulness and self-critical statements.

Signs of depression reported by the examinee include sadness and feelings of despair.

Correct Example: Signs of depression observed during the interview include tearfulness and self-critical statements.

Symptoms of depression reported by the examinee include sadness and feelings of despair.

D   Medical Records

Rule III-D01: When possible, obtain and review relevant medical records, especially recent records and records describing the onset of the injury or illness, and indicate in your report the records that you have reviewed.

Rationale: Examinees are more likely to be cooperative with testing if they perceive that you have taken the time to learn about their background.

You are more likely to reach valid conclusions if you understand the medical context in which your examinees' cognitive problems arise.

Your work will be less vulnerable to critique if you demonstrate thoroughness in reviewing records.

Exceptions or Clarifications: The nature of the referral will often dictate the extent to which records should be reviewed; more thorough review is generally expected in forensic contexts.

Rule III-D02: Do not claim to have reviewed records that you did not actually review.

Rationale: To avoid the embarrassment and other possible negative consequences of being compelled to admit during a deposition or trial that you did not actually review key information that you claimed to have reviewed.

Incorrect Example: Attributing complaints (e.g., headaches and memory problems) entirely to an auto accident when records you claimed to have reviewed indicate that the same complaints were made prior to the accident.

Rule III-D03: When reporting complex medical information, it is generally best to present the information verbatim with quotation marks and to cite your source.

Rationale: This practice will avoid the appearance that you are operating outside the scope of your expertise. Also, in cases in which the medical information is inaccurate or poorly written, the reader will be less likely to attribute the ignorance or sloppiness to you.

Exceptions or Clarifications: In cases in which the error in the quoted information is particularly egregious, you may indicate to your reader that you recognize this by using the term: [sic]. This is generally inserted immediately following the error. Be careful, however, that you do not offend colleagues or referral sources by unnecessarily drawing attention to their errors in this way.

Rule III-D04: Brand names of medications are customarily capitalized, while generic names are not.

Rationale: The brand name is considered a proper noun and is therefore capitalized in the same manner that you would capitalize Pepsi, for example. Generic names are not considered proper nouns and therefore are not capitalized, just as you would not capitalize cola.

Incorrect Example: Ms. Poppins takes Aspirin and prozac.

Correct Example: Ms. Poppins takes aspirin and Prozac.

Exceptions or Clarifications: In order to avoid the necessity of looking up medication names to determine whether they are generic or brand names, it is acceptable to list medications in a columnar format in which each entry in the column is capitalized. For example:

Medications reported by Ms. Poppins include:

Prozac
Aspirin
Valium
Hydrochlorothiazide

E   Medical, Psychiatric, and Substance Exposure History

Rule III-E01: Names of diseases and syndromes are not typically capitalized, but certain words in disease or syndrome names are properly capitalized when they are the surname of the person who first identified the condition, a geographical region associated with the condition, or another term that is customarily capitalized. Acronyms and initialisms, however, are typically capitalized.

Rationale: Standard rules of capitalization.

Incorrect Examples: Alzheimer's Disease
                            alzheimer's disease
                            ptsd

Correct Examples: Alzheimer's disease
PTSD
Legionnaire's disease
West Nile virus

Exceptions or Clarifications: One of the most common mistakes of this type occurs when the writer is accustomed to seeing the disease written in the form of a capitalized initialism or acronym. For example, many writers mistakenly capitalize multiple sclerosis because they are accustomed to seeing the properly capitalized initialism, MS.

One acceptable exception to the capitalization rule explained above is to capitalize mental health disorders when they are listed at the end of a psychological or neuropsychological report as formal diagnoses. There are three rationales for this exception.

The first rationale is that the Diagnostic and Statistical Manual of Mental Disorders has established the convention of capitalizing mental disorders. The second rationale is that capitalization of diagnostic terms at the end of your report may help your reader to more readily identify this important information, although bold font will also help in this regard. The third rationale is that mental disorders are more likely to be viewed by some readers as worthy of attention if formalized by capitalization. For example, a utilization reviewer may be more likely to authorize treatment for "Personality Change Due to Head Trauma" than for "personality change due to head trauma."

Rule III-E02: When describing substance use history, attribute your statements to the source of your information.

Rationale: To avoid allegations of libel.

Incorrect Example: Mr. Smith used heroin almost daily from age 24 to 29.

Correct Example: According to his mother's report during our interview, Mr. Smith used heroin almost daily from age 24 to 29.

Rule III-E03: When gathering history, pay careful attention to medical conditions or potential sources of toxic exposure that might account for your examinee's cognitive impairment.

Rationale: From a medical-legal perspective, it is important to avoid misattribution of causation. From a patient-care perspective, failure to alert medical providers to a correctible cause of cognitive impairment can lead to unnecessary further impairment.

Exceptions or Clarifications: In most cases you will not be able to conclude definitively that the medical condition or toxic exposure is the cause of cognitive decline, but you can still alert medical providers to investigate further.

F   Social History

Rule III-F01: When reporting language background in someone who is not a native speaker of English, note the language that was learned first, the age at which English was learned, and the current pattern of language usage.

Rationale: In order to correctly select and interpret tests, it is essential to understand the examinee's language background.

Incorrect Example: Ms. Lopez speaks both Spanish and English.

Correct Example: Ms. Lopez reported that she first learned Spanish in the home from family members, but began speaking English when she started school at age 5. While growing up, she reportedly spoke English in school and with her friends and siblings, but spoke mostly Spanish with her parents. She stated that she currently speaks mostly English and indicated that her thoughts are typically in English.

Rule III-F02: When reporting on education level, be careful to differentiate between actual graduation from high school and mere entry into 12th grade without graduating or completion of the GED.

Rationale: The criteria established by norms developers dictate how education levels are defined when applying their norms to your patients. For example, some norms developers have not regarded attainment of a GED as equivalent to high school graduation and have not considered mere entry into a grade as equivalent to completion of that grade.

Incorrect Example: Ms. O'Toole reported her highest level of educational attainment as 12th grade.

Correct Example: Ms. O'Toole reported that she dropped out of the 12th grade but later obtained a GED.

Rule III-F03: When reporting education level, be careful to differentiate between post-secondary trade school education and academic college education.

Rationale: Some test norms developers have not counted vocational or trade school training in determining years of education.

Incorrect Example: Giving credit for additional years of education beyond high school to someone who attended truck-driving school or completed an apprenticeship in plumbing, even though both may have involved classroom education, when the norms developer did not count such training when determining years of education.

Correct Example: Giving credit for the highest level of formal academic education achieved according to the criteria established by the norms developer.

Exceptions or Clarifications: At times it may be necessary to use clinical judgment regarding the patient's educational background and clearly state your basis for determination of education level in selecting the appropriate normative comparison group.

Certain situations are quite complex, such as the situation in which a patient has technically graduated from high school, but did so from a special-education program with reduced standards for graduation. In cases such as this, it may be helpful to obtain scores using two different educational comparison groups. For example, it may be most appropriate to compare the patient to others with a regular high school diploma if the evaluation is being conducted to determine suitability for employment in a job requiring 12 years of education. On the other hand, if a conclusion is required regarding whether the patient has suffered a decline in mental ability due to an injury, it may be more appropriate to estimate actual level of premorbid functioning, which may be lower than that of the typical high school graduate.

Rule III-F04: In descriptions of an examinee's work history, names of jobs are not typically capitalized, unless listing a specific job title within an organization or a word that is customarily capitalized.

> *Rationale*: Standard rules of capitalization.

> *Incorrect Examples*: Registered Nurse
> english teacher
> History Teacher
> senior surgical technician II

> *Correct Examples*: registered nurse
> English teacher
> history teacher
> Senior Surgical Technician II

> *Exceptions or Clarifications*: Acronyms and initialisms, such as R.N., are typically capitalized.

Rule III-F05: When reporting a patient's source of disability income, be precise in stating the specific type of income.

> *Rationale*: Precise determination of the type of disability income can help you and readers of your report understand what the patient is receiving, how long the income is expected to last, and what additional benefits might be applied for by the patient or patient's family.

> *Incorrect Example*: He reported receiving disability income.

> *Correct Example*: He reported being on total temporary disability through workers' compensation and said he has recently applied for disability through Social Security.

Rule III-F06: Capitalize sources of funding that are names of specific government or private programs, but do not capitalize generic sources of income.

> *Rationale*: Compliance with standard rules of written expression will facilitate your readers' understanding of your reports.

> *Incorrect Example*: She currently receives social security disability income benefits and no longer receives income from a private Disability Insurance policy.

> *Correct Example*: She currently receives Social Security Disability Income benefits and no longer receives income from a private disability insurance policy.

> *Exceptions or Clarifications*: Acronyms and initialisms are usually capitalized even when the term they represent would not be capitalized if spelled out.

Rule III-F07: When examinees report unusually high premorbid IQ scores, question them carefully and ask for documentation (if available).

> *Rationale*: Examinees may not remember accurately, may inflate scores, may have been misinformed about a score by a family member, or may have taken an "IQ test" (e.g., on the Internet) that is not comparable to traditional IQ measures.

Rule III-F08: When reporting implausible statements made by an examinee or family member, attribute such statements to their source, seek verification, and alert your reader as appropriate to the potential inaccuracy of the information.

> *Rationale*: To avoid appearing gullible and naïve.
>
> *Incorrect Example*: Although currently homeless, he holds a number of patents associated with GPS technology.
>
> *Correct Example*: Although currently homeless, he reported that he holds a number of patents associated with GPS technology. However, his spouse confided that he holds no such patents, and his name was not discovered in an on-line search at USPTO.gov.

Rule III-F09: When gathering information about the examinee's family relationships and living situation, be alert to "red flags" related to possible endangerment to the examinee, children, or others, and respond appropriately if concerns are identified.

> *Rationale*: To fulfill your obligation as a mandated reporter and to decrease the likelihood of harm to others.

Rule III-F10: In gathering history, be alert to psychosocial stressors that might be contributing to your examinee's emotional distress and/or cognitive inefficiency.

> *Rationale*: From a medical-legal perspective, it is important to avoid misattribution of causation. From a patient-care perspective, failure to identify a correctible or treatable cause of emotional distress or cognitive inefficiency can lead to unnecessary further suffering.

Chapter 5
Selecting Tests and Categorizing Performance

Rule IV-01: In selecting a test battery for a particular case, consider these factors:

1. Applicability of tests to the referral question(s)
2. Efficiency of the battery
3. Linguistic, motor, sensory, or other factors that need to be taken into account
4. Availability of demographically appropriate norms

   Rationale: To increase the usefulness and validity of the evaluation.

   Exceptions or Clarifications: Be mindful that there can be advantages to using a standard core battery, especially in forensic contexts.

Rule IV-02: Prior to using descriptive labels such as mild, moderate, and severe, define the labels for your reader, or else accompany each label with a meaningful numerical score.

   Rationale: To promote common understanding, as research has revealed lack of consensus among professionals regarding what is meant by such terms (e.g., Guilmette T. J., Hagan, L. D.,& Giuliano, A. J., 2008, Assigning qualitative descriptions to test scores in neuropsychology: Forensic implications, *Clinical Neuropsychology*, 122–139; Wanlass, R. L., Reutter, S. L., & Kline, A.E., 1992, Communication among rehabilitation staff: "Mild," "moderate," or "severe" deficits? *Archives Physical Medicine Rehabilitation*, 477–481).

   Incorrect Example: She demonstrated a mild deficit in delayed visual recall.

   Correct Examples:

   <u>*SYSTEM FOR CATEGORIZING SCORES*</u>: On tests for which standardized scores (e.g., T-scores or percentiles) are available, a classification system is applied such that scores one standard deviation or more below the mean (less than or equal to the 16th percentile) are considered to fall in the <u>mild</u> deficit range. Scores two or more standard deviations below the mean (less than or equal to the 2nd percentile) are considered to fall in the <u>moderate</u> deficit range. Scores three or more standard deviations below the mean (less than or equal to the 0.1 percentile) are considered to fall in the <u>severe</u> deficit range. Scores that are above the 16th percentile but not greater than the 25th percentile are designated as falling in the <u>low average</u> range. Scores falling above the 25th percentile and below the 75th percentile are classified as <u>average</u>. Scores ranging from the 75th percentile to just below the 84th

percentile are categorized as <u>high average</u>. Scores within this broad band from just above the 16th percentile to just below the 84th percentile are considered <u>within normal limits</u>.

Scores falling far above average are labeled as <u>superior</u> (greater than or equal to the 84th percentile), <u>very superior</u> (greater than or equal to the 98th percentile), or <u>exceptional</u> (greater than or equal to the 99.9th percentile), depending upon whether they are one, two, or three standard deviations above the mean.

She scored in the mild deficit range (5th %ile).

Exceptions or Clarifications: Bear in mind that the labeling system included in the example above is just one of many possible ways of categorizing scores; the neuropsychology profession has yet to agree on a standard labeling system.

Rule IV-03: If it is ever necessary or useful to describe a specific test performance with an alternate labeling system, make it clear to the reader that you are doing so.

Rationale: To avoid confusing the reader or appearing inconsistent.

Incorrect Example: This Full Scale IQ of 75 falls at the 5th %ile and in the borderline range.

Correct Example: This Full Scale IQ of 75 falls at the 5th %ile and in the mild deficit range according to the labeling system applied throughout this report. For the purpose of communication with school district personnel who are more accustomed to the Wechsler system for categorizing scores, this IQ is in the "borderline" range according to the Wechsler system.

Rule IV-04: Apply common sense to avoid being overly rigid or simplistic regarding performance categories.

Rationale: To increase the validity and utility of your report.

Incorrect Example: While her immediate story recall tested in the normal range (17th%ile), Ms. Cohen performed worse on delayed story recall, falling in the mild deficit range (15th%ile).

Correct Example: Ms. Cohen's story recall performance was similar for both immediate recall (17th%ile) and delayed recall (15th%ile).

Chapter 6
Testing, Interpreting, and Reporting Results

A   Validity

Rule V-A01: Determine adequacy of visual acuity (i.e., near vision), visual fields, and visual attention before administering tests that require reading or other vision-related functions. If there are correctible problems, provide appropriate corrections. If there are problems that cannot be corrected, take vision-related limitations into account in test selection and interpretation.

> *Rationale*: To make sure that you are validly measuring the function that you intend to measure.
>
> *Incorrect Example*: Obtaining a low premorbid IQ estimate on the reading task because of vision problems that interfere with reading of words that could have been recognized if vision correction (e.g., use of glasses) or larger print had been provided.
>
> *Correct Example*: Making sure that vision is adequately corrected or that test stimuli are sufficiently large to permit valid assessment.

Rule V-A02: Encourage cooperation and effort from test subjects, and verify cooperation and effort through use of validity tests.

> *Rationale*: Some examinees are influenced by external incentives to perform poorly, while others may not fully cooperate because they resent being compelled to go through testing or simply do not possess high achievement motivation as it pertains to testing.
>
> *Incorrect Example*: Assuming all subjects are fully cooperative, not encouraging effort, and not verifying test validity.
>
> *Correct Example*: Encouraging effort and verifying test validity.
>
> *Exceptions or Clarifications*: Consider in some contexts cautioning the subject that your battery will include assessment of effort, but be careful not to divulge how it is being assessed or by what measures.

R.L. Wanlass, *The Neuropsychology Toolkit: Guidelines, Formats, and Language,*
DOI 10.1007/ 978-1-4614-1882-5_6, © Springer Science+Business Media, LLC 2012

Rule V-A03: Assess validity with extra thoroughness in cases in which clear external incentives for submaximal performance are evident.

> *Rationale*: To increase the likelihood of correctly identifying the degree of cooperation and effort on testing.

> *Incorrect Example*: Passing performance on the RFIT indicates good effort and cooperation with testing for the effects of Mr. Johnson's fall from the collapsing hotel balcony.

> *Correct Example*: Passing performance on the WMT, TOMM, and three embedded measures indicates good effort and cooperation with testing for the effects of Mr. Johnson's fall from the collapsing hotel balcony.

> *Exceptions or Clarifications*: In certain contexts, the actual names of the validity measures are omitted from the report by some experts to protect test security.

Rule V-A04: Be aware of the examinee's current medications and comment on the potential impact of the medications on cognition.

> *Rationale*: Many medications may impact cognition.

> *Exceptions or Clarifications*: Sometimes, medications affect cognition, but test results are still considered reflective of typical daily functioning if the examinee takes the medication on an ongoing basis.

B   Intellectual and Problem-Solving Ability

Rule V-B01: When estimating premorbid IQ based on reading ability, account for the presence of dyslexia and limited cultural/linguistic/educational exposure.

> *Rationale*: To avoid potentially harmful misinterpretation of results (e.g., smaller personal injury settlement based upon an incorrect conclusion about below-normal pre-injury intellectual ability).

> *Incorrect Example*: Mr. Chin, a dyslexic recent immigrant from China, obtained a very low score on the TOPF reading task, indicating below-average pre-injury intelligence.

> *Correct Example*: Because of his dyslexia and cultural/linguistic background, Mr. Chin's low score on the TOPF is not sufficient basis for assuming below-average premorbid intelligence.

Rule V-B02: In estimating premorbid IQ based on demographics, be mindful of factors other than intelligence that might limit educational or occupational achievement, including:

1. current youth
2. youth at the time of injury
3. unusual restrictions on opportunities (e.g., economic or geographical limitations)

> *Rationale*: To avoid interpretation errors stemming from inaccurate premorbid IQ estimates.

Rule V-B03: In estimating premorbid IQ through use of reading tests (e.g., WTAR or TOPF), be mindful of floor and ceiling restrictions affecting persons at IQ extremes.

Rationale: To avoid interpretation errors stemming from inaccurate premorbid IQ estimates.

Rule V-B04: Do not use the word "problem" when describing difficulty the examinee had with problem-solving tasks.

Rationale: To decrease the chance of reader confusion.

Incorrect Example: He demonstrated problems with problem-solving.

Correct Example: He demonstrated difficulty with problem-solving.

Rule V-B05: In selecting specific IQ subtests to administer when time is limited, give preference to subtests that:

1. contribute to relevant indices (e.g., processing speed, working memory)
2. are less vulnerable to test confounds (e.g., sensory, motor, linguistic) for that particular examinee
3. assess functions of most clinical relevance to that particular examinee
4. are time efficient

Rationale: To maximize evaluation efficiency, relevance, and validity.

Rule V-B06: Be mindful of the limited sensitivity of IQ scores to the cognitive sequelae of many neurological conditions (e.g., traumatic brain injury).

Rationale: To reduce the likelihood of minimizing legitimate cognitive deficits.

Incorrect Example: Concluding absence of cognitive sequelae of a traumatic brain injury on the basis of a normal IQ.

Correct Example: Taking into account other evidence from tests that are more sensitive to cognitive sequelae of neurological conditions.

Exceptions or Clarifications: Some IQ subtests (e.g., digit-symbol substitution tasks) are more sensitive than others to cognitive sequelae of neurological conditions.

C   Processing Speed

Rule V-C01: Be careful about interpreting poor Trails A performance as reflective of slow mental processing when the Trails B score is not also low.

Rationale: To make sure that interpretations are valid and consistent with common sense analysis.

Exceptions or Clarifications: Be alert to other possible explanations, besides slow mental processing for poor Trails A performance (e.g., hand covering a number preventing progression for several seconds).

Rule V-C02: In assessing mental processing speed, be mindful of potential confounds associated with the examinee's motor or speech limitations.

> *Rationale*: To increase accuracy of test interpretation.
>
> *Incorrect Example*: Assessing processing speed based on written or other motor output in a person with a physical restriction on mobility or dexterity and not taking this confound into account.
>
> *Correct Example*: Attempting to select tests that minimize the presence of confounds and taking unavoidable confounds into account in interpretation.

Rule V-C03: When interpreting speed performance on cancellation tasks, pay attention to accuracy.

> *Rationale*: To avoid giving too much credit for speed when accuracy is poor, or to avoid over-interpretation of a poor speed score when the examinee has chosen to sacrifice speed for the sake of extreme precision.

D Mental Control

Rule V-D01: If using the term "executive functioning," provide your reader with a description of the specific aspects of executive functioning to which you are referring and recognize the limitations of structured tests alone as indicators of executive functioning.

> *Rationale*: To facilitate accurate understanding by your readers, as this term is not consistently conceptualized and operationally defined by professionals and is generally not well understood by lay people.
>
> *Incorrect Example*: Impaired executive functioning was evident in Mr. Singh's poor test results.
>
> *Correct Example*: Dr. Fong's referral requested that we assess Mr. Singh's executive functioning. This term is generally used to refer to higher-order cognitive skills involved in the planning and organization of goal-directed activity, as well as the self-monitoring of progress and flexible adjustment of strategies in the pursuit of goals. Observations of Mr. Singh's approach to block-design and figure-drawing tasks revealed inadequate planning, organization, and self-monitoring. These observations are consistent with reports by family members and work supervisors that Mr. Singh has been sloppier in his work and less able to successfully plan out, organize, and follow through on projects since his traumatic brain injury. In the absence of other explanatory factors for these changes in behavior (e.g., depression, medication side-effects, substance abuse), it does appear that Mr. Singh's executive functioning has been compromised.

E   Learning and Memory

Rule V-E01: In assessing memory, be mindful of the potential for practice effect from prior exposure to the same memory stimuli.

Rationale: To increase the validity of test results.

Incorrect Example: Re-administering the same story memory test a week after previous testing and not acknowledging the likely practice effect.

Correct Example: Attempting to find an appropriate alternate story memory task, or at least acknowledging the likely practice effect.

Rule V-E02: Pay attention to the pattern of performance on memory tasks to help differentiate between retention and retrieval.

Rationale: To elucidate strengths and weaknesses in order to facilitate differential diagnosis and identification of appropriate compensatory strategies.

Incorrect Example: On a verbal list-learning task, Ms. Ray demonstrated impaired free recall, but normal performance on a recognition task.

Correct Example: On a verbal list-learning task, Ms. Ray demonstrated impaired free recall, but normal performance on a recognition task. This pattern of performance indicates that Ms. Ray has difficulty retrieving and freely recalling newly acquired verbal information, but with cues is able to correctly recognize this information. This shows that she is able to retain new information.

Rule V-E03: When assessing visual memory, be careful to take into account non-memory factors that affect reproduction of visual stimuli.

Rationale: To increase interpretation accuracy.

Incorrect Example: Concluding evidence of impaired visual memory from a poor score on a complex design recall task when the copy performance is comparably poor.

F   Communication

Rule V-F01: Include observations on volume, articulation, speed, prosody, or any other aspects of communication that are noteworthy but not necessarily assessed well by standardized tests.

Rationale: To provide the reader with a more complete picture of the examinee's communication functioning.

Rule V-F02: In cases in which listening comprehension is intact for shorter instructions, but not for longer instructions, pay attention to memory test performance to try to differentiate between poor memory and receptive aphasia.

> *Rationale*: To avoid mislabeling a patient as aphasic when the impaired performance is actually due to poor memory.
>
> *Exceptions or Clarifications*: Sometimes both problems are present, and sometimes receptive aphasia will make it more difficult to accurately assess memory.

G Motor Functions

Rule V-G01: Do not put medically fragile patients, or yourself, at risk by having them perform physically strenuous or hazardous activities.

> *Rationale*: Avoidance of harm to the patient and avoidance of liability.
>
> *Incorrect Examples*: Administering a grip strength test to an elderly man recovering from carpal tunnel surgery, heart attack, and aneurysm rupture.
>
> Assessing balance in a morbidly obese woman with Ménière's disease and severe osteoporosis.

Rule V-G02: Include observations about ambulation, for example, speed, balance, or need for assistive device.

> *Rationale*: To provide the reader with a more complete picture of the patient's motor functioning beyond the areas typically assessed by neuropsychological tests.

H Visual-Spatial Functions

Rule V-H01: Be careful about interpreting poor Trails A performance as reflective of poor visual scanning when the Trails B score is not also low.

> *Rationale*: To make sure that interpretations are valid and consistent with common sense analysis.
>
> *Exceptions or Clarifications*: Be alert to other possible explanations, besides slow visual scanning for poor Trails A performance (e.g., hand covering a number preventing progression for several seconds).

Rule V-H02: Be mindful of the distinction between visual neglect (an attentional problem) and visual field loss (a perceptual problem).

> *Rationale*: To accurately describe the examinee's functioning.
>
> *Exceptions or Clarifications*: Some examinees have both field loss and neglect.

Rule V-H03: When interpreting accuracy of performance on cancellation tasks, pay attention to speed.

> *Rationale*: To avoid giving too much credit for accuracy when speed is poor, or to avoid over-interpretation of a poor accuracy score when the examinee has chosen to sacrifice accuracy for the sake of extreme speed.

I   Olfactory Perception

Rule V-I01: In assessing smell with scratch-and-sniff or similar stimuli, verify the freshness of each scent

> *Rationale*: To reduce the likelihood of over-pathologizing.

Rule V-I02: In assessing smell, be mindful of factors other than brain injury that might affect smell, such as nasal congestion from a cold or allergies.

> *Rationale*: To reduce the likelihood of over-pathologizing.

J   Mental Status and Psychological Adjustment

Rule V-J01: Assess for suicidal thoughts, plan, and intent, and be sure to document in your report that you have done so.

> *Rationale*: To make certain that you do not miss important clinical information and to protect yourself from liability.

> *Exceptions or Clarifications*: If risk factors are identified, document in detail how you assessed and dealt with them.

Rule V-J02: In describing a patient's performance at answering safety judgment questions, bear in mind the limitations of such tests.

> *Rationale*: Some patients may be able to answer such questions appropriately, but still present a serious safety risk without supervision because of a tendency to act impulsively and/ or failure to recognize deficits (e.g., visual neglect) that could put them at risk.

> *Incorrect Example*: Despite Mr. Gage's large bi-frontal lesions, safety judgment is fully intact as demonstrated by superior performance (85%ile) on the NAB Judgment subtest. Thus, he no longer appears in need of supervision.

> *Correct Example*: Mr. Gage performed in the superior range (85%ile) when asked to respond to safety judgment questions on the NAB Judgment subtest. However, as is common for persons with large bi-frontal injuries, he demonstrated several instances of impulsivity during testing, and his family provided several more examples. In addition, he has minimal recognition of his visual neglect problem. Thus, the overall clinical picture suggests serious safety concerns and need for continued close supervision.

Chapter 7
Reporting Conclusions, Diagnoses, and Recommendations

Rule VI-01: In drawing conclusions about the examinee's condition, be mindful of the distinction between "impairment," which implies that there has been a decline from a previous level of functioning, and "deficit," which implies only that ability in that particular domain is lacking.

> *Rationale*: To communicate more clearly regarding both level of functioning and changes in level of functioning.

> *Exceptions or Clarifications*: An examinee might exhibit **impairment** relative to a high premorbid level of functioning in a certain domain and yet still score in the normal or better range and, therefore, not exhibit a **deficit** in that domain.

> Another examinee might score below the normal range in a certain domain, thereby exhibiting a **deficit**, and yet not show **impairment** if the evidence indicates that this was always an area of weakness (and that functioning in this domain has not worsened since the injury or illness).

Rule VI-02: The basis of any diagnosis should be clearly established in your report of history, patient self-report, collateral information, observations, and test results so that a knowledgeable reader would not be surprised by your diagnostic decision.

> *Rationale*: This practice helps to make sure that you think clearly about your diagnostic decision and helps to communicate to your reader that you have done so.

Rule VI-03: When diagnosing dementia in a case in which the dementia is not expected to be progressive (e.g., dementia due to head trauma), make certain that your written report and feedback clearly indicate that you are not implying that the condition is expected to progress.

> *Rationale*: Patients and family members, as well as many professionals, are inclined to infer from the term "dementia" that you are predicting a progressive decline in cognitive functioning. Explanation can prevent unnecessary worry.

R.L. Wanlass, *The Neuropsychology Toolkit: Guidelines, Formats, and Language,*   33
DOI 10.1007/ 978-1-4614-1882-5_7, © Springer Science+Business Media, LLC 2012

Incorrect Example: Diagnostically, Mr. McDonald's condition can be best categorized as dementia due to head trauma.

Correct Example: Diagnostically, Mr. McDonald's condition can be best categorized as dementia due to head trauma. It is important to point out, however, that the use of the diagnostic term "dementia" in this case does not imply a progressive condition.

Exceptions or Clarifications: Be mindful of research suggesting increased likelihood and/or earlier onset of progressive dementia in some who have sustained traumatic brain injury.

Rule VI-04: The recommendation section of your report is often potentially its most valuable component and, therefore, deserves thorough deliberation and research.

Rationale: To improve report utility and increase the likelihood of subsequent referrals.

Incorrect Example: It is recommended that Ms. Oh be referred for psychotherapy.

Correct Example: It is recommended that Ms. Oh be referred for 10 sessions of individual cognitive-behavioral psychotherapy for her mildly depressed mood. Because of her type of insurance, she or her family will need to contact Acme Behavioral Health (800-555-5555) for a referral. I have advised them to do so and encouraged them to request a psychotherapist experienced with adjustment issues related to disability. Ms. Oh and her family agreed to follow through on this recommendation.

Rule VI-05: In giving oral feedback on test results to examinees, family members, or others who do not share your training and vocabulary proficiency, be careful to communicate with understandable language and pause frequently to invite questions and verify understanding.

Rationale: To increase the utility of feedback.

Chapter 8
Writing Effectively

This section addresses some of the most common writing errors I see in neuropsychological reports, but contains only a small portion of the rules of good writing found in more general writing handbooks. The reader is encouraged to consult such handbooks as needed for guidance regarding writing rules not addressed here. Bear in mind that the "rules" of writing may vary somewhat from one handbook to another.

Rule VII-01: Educational degrees are capitalized when listed in the form of an initialism (e.g., M.S.), but not when spelled out (e.g., master's degree).

> *Rationale*: Compliance with standard rules of capitalization contributes to the professional appearance of your reports.
>
> *Incorrect Examples*: She has a Master's in Science degree.
>
> She has an m.s. degree.
>
> *Correct Examples*: She has a master's in science degree.
>
> She has an M.S. degree.

Rule VII-02: In a compound sentence in which the two parts are separated by the conjunction "and" or "but," insert a comma before the conjunction. (Compound sentences are composed of two or more units, each of which has both a subject and a verb and could stand alone as a complete sentence).

> *Rationale*: Compliance with standard rules of punctuation contributes to the professional appearance of your reports.
>
> *Incorrect Examples*: He performed the writing task rather hastily and he made numerous errors in punctuation and spelling.
>
> He performed the writing task rather hastily, and made numerous errors.
>
> *Correct Examples*: He performed the writing task rather hastily, and he made numerous errors.
>
> He performed the writing task rather hastily and made numerous errors.

R.L. Wanlass, *The Neuropsychology Toolkit: Guidelines, Formats, and Language,*
DOI 10.1007/ 978-1-4614-1882-5_8, © Springer Science+Business Media, LLC 2012

Exceptions or Clarifications: When a compound sentence is very short, the comma may be omitted.

When each unit does not have its own subject, then you generally should not insert a comma before "and," but may insert a comma before "but" to indicate to the reader the slight pause that normally precedes "but" in this context (as in this sentence).

Rule VII-03: Use the terms "e.g." (meaning "for example") and "i.e." (meaning "that is") correctly, and insert a comma after them.

Rationale: Compliance with standard rules of written expression will facilitate your readers' understanding of your reports.

Incorrect Example: He has tried several antidepressants (i.e. Prozac).

Correct Example: He has tried several antidepressants (e.g., Prozac).

Exceptions or Clarifications: Some scientific journals have adopted a policy of saving space by reducing punctuation such as the comma following e.g., but clinical reports are generally best understood if they follow more conventional writing style.

Rule VII-04: When stating that somebody "reported" something, precede what was reported by the word "that" if you are not directly quoting the informant and if the information you are conveying in your sentence has both a subject and a verb.

Rationale: This guideline will facilitate your reader's understanding of your reports.

Incorrect Example: He reported his wife has been arrested.

Correct Examples: He reported that his wife has been arrested.

He reported being hungry.

Exceptions or Clarifications: No one will consider you a poor writer for not following this particular suggestion, but it does seem to facilitate reader comprehension. The reason for potential confusion is that when reading words like "he reported" followed immediately by words like "his wife," your reader is momentarily uncertain as to whether to think that "he" filed some report against his wife or simply related to you some information about her.

Rule VII-05: Compound adjectives are hyphenated when they precede the word that they modify, but not when they follow it.

Rationale: Compliance with standard rules of written expression will facilitate your readers' understanding of your reports.

Incorrect Examples: She has a 17 year old son.
                      Her son is 17-years-old.

Correct Examples: She has a 17-year-old son.
                    Her son is 17 years old.

Rule VII-06: The word "however" is technically not a conjunction and should not be used interchangeably with the word "but" unless you precede it with a semi-colon (;) and follow it with a comma.

Rationale: Compliance with standard rules of written expression will facilitate your readers' understanding of your reports.

Incorrect Example: He reported difficulty with concentration, however he was able to perform normally on all concentration tasks.

Correct Examples: He reported difficulty with concentration; however, he was able to perform normally on all concentration tasks.

He reported difficulty with concentration, but he was able to perform normally on all concentration tasks.

Rule VII-07: To write good reports, write well, including proper use of "good" (as an adjective that answers the question "what kind of?") and "well" (as an adverb that answers the question "how?").

Rationale: Adherence to conventions of English language usage facilitates reader understanding and conveys an image of professionalism.

Incorrect Example: Drawing tasks were performed good, with well attention to detail.

Correct Example: Drawing tasks were performed well, with good attention to detail.

Exceptions or Clarifications: It is, however, correct in some situations to describe a person as doing good, for example when the person is performing acts of charity.

Rule VII-08: Use "that" to introduce a phrase or clause containing information essential to understanding the main point of the sentence. Use "which" to introduce a nonessential phrase or clause, and set this nonessential, or parenthetical, phrase or clause off with commas.

Rationale: Adherence to this guideline will facilitate reader understanding by alerting them to the type of information conveyed within the phrase or clause.

Incorrect Examples: He exhibited difficulty on tasks **which** required manual dexterity.

He exhibited difficulty on manual dexterity tasks, **that** is consistent with his self-reported difficulty with using small tools.

Correct Examples: He exhibited difficulty on tasks **that** required manual dexterity.

He exhibited difficulty on manual dexterity tasks, **which** is consistent with his self-reported difficulty with using small tools.

Exceptions or Clarifications: "Nonessential" does not mean "irrelevant," as irrelevant information should not be included in the report at all.

Some grammar authorities have relaxed this rule to permit use of "which" to introduce essential information if this does not cause confusion to the reader.

Rule VII-09: Commas precede the year when listing an exact date and also follow the year when the sentence continues beyond the year.

Rationale: Adherence to conventions of English language punctuation enhances the professional appearance of your reports.

Incorrect Example: She was admitted to the hospital on October 12, 2010 and discharged a week later.

Correct Example: She was admitted to the hospital on October 12, 2010, and discharged a week later.

Exceptions or Clarifications: The comma rule does not apply when dates are listed in abbreviated formats such as 11/11/2011.

Rule VII-10: Commas precede the listing of a professional degree after a person's name and also follow the degree when the sentence continues beyond the degree.

Rationale: Adherence to conventions of English language punctuation enhances the professional appearance of your reports.

Incorrect Examples: He was referred to Juan Lopez M.D. for psychiatric evaluation.

He was referred to Juan Lopez M.D.

Correct Examples: He was referred to Juan Lopez, M.D., for psychiatric evaluation.

He was referred to Juan Lopez, M.D.

Rule VII-11: When listing items in a series, use parallel construction, which means employing the same grammatical form for each item.

Rationale: To facilitate reader comprehension and enhance the professional image conveyed by your writing.

Incorrect Example: She listened carefully, answered concisely, and was clear in her enunciation.

Correct Example: She listened carefully, answered concisely, and enunciated clearly.

Rule VII-12: When using an introductory phrase or clause longer than a few words, separate it from the remainder of the sentence with a comma.

Rationale: The comma helps your reader recognize the transition from introductory phrase or clause to the main part of the sentence and shows where a slight pause would occur if the sentence were read aloud.

Incorrect Example: When she experienced a scheduling conflict with the examiner she displayed sound judgment.

Correct Example: When she experienced a scheduling conflict with the examiner, she displayed sound judgment.

Rule VII-13: Add a zero before a number that starts with a decimal point.

Rationale: To reduce the possibility of cases in which the decimal is omitted or not clearly seen and to comply with Joint Commission guidelines.

Incorrect Example: .9%ile

Correct Example: 0.9%ile

Rule VII-14: Alert the reader to the presence of unexpected inconsistency by using terms like "however," "but," and "while."

> *Rationale*: To facilitate reader understanding.
>
> *Incorrect Example*: Her safety judgment tested in the superior range, and she demonstrated limited deficit awareness.
>
> *Correct Examples*: Her safety judgment tested in the superior range, but she demonstrated limited deficit awareness.
>
> Her safety judgment tested in the superior range. However, she demonstrated limited deficit awareness.
>
> While her safety judgment tested in the superior range, she demonstrated limited deficit awareness.

Rule VII-15: Use present verb tense to describe an activity or state that is ongoing and past verb tense to describe an activity or state that occurred at one point in the past but cannot be assumed to be ongoing.

> *Rationale*: To facilitate reader comprehension by communicating more accurately.
>
> *Incorrect Examples*: He speaks frequently about his anger at the person who caused his injury.
>
> She was tall.
>
> *Correct Examples*: He spoke frequently about his anger at the person who caused his injury.
>
> She is tall.

Rule VII-16: Use the appropriate verb form.

> *Rationale*: Clarity of communication.
>
> *Incorrect Example*: As a child he would have difficulty sitting still.
>
> *Correct Example*: As a child he had difficulty sitting still.

Rule VII-17: Correctly distinguish between "affect" and "effect." As a noun in neuropsychological reports, "affect" refers to observable emotion, while as a verb it most often means to have an influence upon. "Effect" as a noun most often refers to the result of a cause, while as a verb it means to accomplish or put into operation.

> *Rationale*: Using words as they are conventionally defined facilitates communication.
>
> *Incorrect Example*: The sad movie effected him as evidenced by his tearful effect.
>
> *Correct Example*: The sad movie affected him as evidenced by his tearful affect.
>
> *Exceptions or Clarifications*: Other definitions of these terms exist, but are less commonly used in neuropsychological and psychological reports.

Rule VII-18: In reporting temporal order of occurrences, do not, through imprecise writing, state or imply that an event or condition occurred or started before it actually did.

>   *Rationale*: To facilitate reader understanding.
>
>   *Incorrect Examples*: Prior to his current injury, he denied any pre-existing memory problems.
>
>   Since her injury five years ago, she reported progressive deterioration in her memory.
>
>   *Correct Examples*: He denied having any pre-injury memory problems.
>
>   She reported noticing progressive deterioration in her memory since her injury five years ago.
>
>   *Exceptions or Clarifications*: In the first incorrect example, we most likely do not really know what he denied prior to his injury. In the second incorrect example, it is unlikely that she immediately began reporting progressive deterioration after her injury since it probably took a while to notice the progression.

Rule VII-19: Use a comma to indicate the point in the sentence at which a reader would appropriately pause to add clarity.

>   *Rationale*: To increase the ease with which your reader can comprehend what you are trying to communicate.
>
>   *Incorrect Example*: Ms. Alvarez's visual-spatial ability tested in the unimpaired range with a relative strength in her figure copy.
>
>   *Correct Example*: Ms. Alvarez's visual-spatial ability tested in the unimpaired range, with a relative strength in her figure copy.
>
>   *Exceptions or Clarifications*: If you do not have a good "ear" for sensing when a pause is appropriate, this method may not work well for you.

Rule VII-20: Use singular verb form when the subject of your sentence or clause is singular, and use plural verb form when the subject of your sentence or clause is plural.

>   *Rationale*: To facilitate reader understanding.
>
>   *Incorrect Example*: His performance on verbal and visual learning and memory tasks indicate that his ability to retrieve facts and images improve with contextual cues.
>
>   *Correct Example*: His performance on verbal and visual learning and memory tasks indicates that his ability to retrieve facts and images improves with contextual cues.
>
>   *Exceptions or Clarifications*: When the subject and verb are separated by several words, errors in subject-verb agreement are more common. In such cases, mentally subtracting out these extraneous words will help you correctly match the subject and verb.

Chapter 9
Controlling Quality

Rule VIII-01: Develop systems to ensure that you follow through on commitments and obligations made in the course of the evaluation process.

> *Rationale*: Failure to follow through on commitments or obligations will result in your being trusted less by patients, supervisors, and referral sources and can, in some circumstances, result in harm to the patient or failure to obtain reimbursement.

> *Incorrect Example*: Making a commitment or undertaking a multi-step obligation but not writing a note to yourself, using a checklist, or implementing some other strategy to ensure follow-through, with the result that the commitment or obligation is not fulfilled.

> *Correct Example*: Writing notes to yourself in your appointment book or using some other reminder system every time you agree to perform a task and using checklists to make sure you accomplish each step of multi-step obligations.

> *Exceptions or Clarifications*: If the reminder system you have in place is insufficient, figure out where the breakdowns tend to occur and then modify or replace your system.

Rule VIII-02: Re-check all mathematical calculations at least once.

> *Rationale*: Errors in mathematical calculations lead to inaccurate test interpretations and recommendations, which can result in harmful outcomes for patients. In addition, errors may be discovered by others, including attorneys who hire other professionals to review your work. Your work on the particular case may be discredited, your reputation and future stream of referrals may be damaged, and you may be subject to a licensure board complaint and/or malpractice action.

> *Incorrect Example*: Totaling raw scores just once and trusting that you have done so accurately.

> *Correct Example*: Totaling raw scores once from top to bottom, writing down the obtained score, checking your addition by totaling the numbers again going from bottom to top or using a calculator, and then comparing the two results to make sure they are the same.

> *Exceptions or Clarifications*: If your math skills prove untrustworthy, triple check your calculations, use a calculator, and/or have someone else check your work.

R.L. Wanlass, *The Neuropsychology Toolkit: Guidelines, Formats, and Language*,
DOI 10.1007/ 978-1-4614-1882-5_9, © Springer Science+Business Media, LLC 2012

Rule VIII-03: Apply common sense to make certain that each test score is consistent with the patient's clinical history and presentation and with other related test data. If any discrepancies are found, look for possible explanations such as incorrect administration or scoring.

> *Rationale*: Unexpected or anomalous findings are often indicative of examiner error.

> *Incorrect Example*: Failing to question a score that indicates a strength or weakness that is inconsistent with other evidence.

> *Correct Example*: Identifying unexpected or anomalous scores and carefully verifying that the test procedure was administered and scored correctly and that appropriate normative data were used.

> *Exceptions or Clarifications*: Sometimes unexpected or anomalous scores are a result of a change in the patient's physical or emotional state, and so it is also important to question the patient when such an unexpected or anomalous score is identified.

Rule VIII-04: Eliminate any actual contradictions and explain any apparent contradictions in your report.

> *Rationale*: Actual contradictions indicate failure in your logical analysis and require correction in order to ensure that your conclusions and recommendations are reasonable.

> *Incorrect Example*: He acknowledged being more irritable and less interested in social activity, but did not score in the depressed range on a depression scale and did not outwardly appear depressed. Thus, there is no evidence of depression.

> *Correct Example*: He acknowledged being more irritable and less interested in social activity, but did not score in the depressed range on a depression scale and did not outwardly appear depressed. Thus, while acknowledging some irritability and reduced social interest, @ does not meet criteria for a diagnosis of clinical depression.

> *Exceptions or Clarifications*: Because of the high working memory demand involved in searching for contradictions, it is wise to do a separate re-reading of your report with this as your only goal.

> Careless use of absolute terms (e.g., all, none, always, never) increases the likelihood of a contradiction occurring in your report.

Rule VIII-05: Use the spelling and grammar check features of your word processor to identify and correct spelling and grammar errors.

> *Rationale*: Poor spelling and grammar can undermine your credibility.

> *Exceptions or Clarifications*: Spelling check glossaries are limited, and it is helpful to add technical terms to your glossary once you have verified the correct spelling.

> Grammar check capability is still somewhat primitive, so your own writing knowledge is often necessary to determine whether to accept recommended changes.

Rule VIII-06: When editing your report, remove redundant, irrelevant, and otherwise extraneous words.

> *Rationale*: Your writing will be more clearly understood and will require less reading time.
>
> *Incorrect Examples*: He performed in the mild deficit range of performance on most measures of working memory that were administered.
>
> His father, a Gulf War veteran, drove him to the evaluation.
>
> She was referred for evaluation by Dr. Kobayashi in order to evaluate her current cognition and emotional status.
>
> *Correct Examples*: He performed in the mild deficit range on most working memory measures.
>
> His father drove him to the evaluation.
>
> She was referred by Dr. Kobayashi for evaluation of her current cognition and emotional status.
>
> *Exceptions or Clarifications*: The most important information is appropriately repeated in the summary and conclusions section(s) of the report.
>
> Elaboration or repetition is sometimes useful for emphasis of important points.

Rule VIII-07: Before finalizing a report, re-read it several times, each time from the perspective of a different potential reader (e.g., referring physician, another neuro-psychologist, attorney, patient, family members of patient), and make appropriate revisions.

> *Rationale*: To increase the likelihood of your report being understood by and of value to potential readers, as well as to strengthen areas that might be subject to critique.

Rule VIII-08: When using normative tables to obtain scores, always carefully read the overall title of the table and the headings for each column and row.

> *Rationale*: To make certain that you are using the appropriate norms (e.g., correct gender, age, education), and that you understand the type of scores being used (e.g., raw scores, T scores, percentile) and the direction of scoring (i.e., whether higher scores indicative of better or worse performance).

Rule VIII-09: Make extra effort to record verbatim your examinee's incorrect or incomplete oral responses to test questions.

> *Rationale*: Examples of what the examinee said are sometimes useful in explaining conclusions that the examinee is deficient in some area (e.g., safety judgment). In contrast, for the sake of efficiency, it is not always necessary to record responses that clearly receive full credit.

Exceptions or Clarifications: The nature of the evaluation often determines the thoroughness with which verbatim responses should be recorded, with forensic evaluations generally calling for more thoroughness to allow for another expert to examine your scoring.

Rule VIII-10: When quoting a statement, put inside the quotation marks exactly what was said by the person you are quoting.

Rationale: To maintain credibility by being as accurate as possible.

Incorrect Example: Mr. Jones reported that he has "totally lost control of his temper since his injury."

Correct Examples: Mr. Jones reported that he has "totally lost control" of his temper since his injury.

Mr. Jones reported that he has "totally lost control of [his] temper since [his] injury."

Exceptions or Clarifications: If words do need to be modified for clarity, then put the modification inside of brackets as shown immediately above.

Rule VIII-11: Use appropriate caution and clarification when interpreting scores from tests whose norms are not normally distributed.

Rationale: To avoid providing misleading information to your reader.

Incorrect Example: Ms. Abdullah's listening comprehension tested in the moderate deficit range on the Complex Ideational Material Test (raw score = 9/12; T = 30; %ile = 2).

Correct Example: Ms. Abdullah's listening comprehension tested in the moderate deficit range on the Complex Ideational Material Test (raw score = 9/12; T = 30; %ile = 2). However, during interview and testing she showed the ability to understand basic questions and to follow one- and two-step commands.

Exceptions or Clarifications: In the example above, the low T score and percentile require clarification to prevent the reader from assuming that listening comprehension is worse than it really is.

Rule VIII-12: Never "recycle" an old report to use on a new patient.

Rationale: To avoid inadvertent inclusion of incorrect information (e.g., another patient's name, incorrect scores, wrong gender reference) that could result in harm to the patient or the appearance of sloppy work.

Exceptions or Clarifications: If there are specific phrases you wish to save for use in subsequent reports, first remove all gender-specific pronouns, names, scores, and any other wording that might not be applicable to all future patients for whom you might use these phrases.

Chapter 10
Post-Test

On the pages that follow, you will find a post-test on which you can demonstrate what you have learned by reading the guidelines above.

Please take a half hour to complete this post-test.

R.L. Wanlass, *The Neuropsychology Toolkit: Guidelines, Formats, and Language,*
DOI 10.1007/ 978-1-4614-1882-5_10, © Springer Science+Business Media, LLC 2012

Glasscow Comma Scale Post-Test

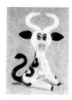

This brief report contains more than 60 errors reflecting limitations in psychological and medical knowledge, writing ability, and common sense. Please correct as many errors (including errors of both commission and omission) as you can in the next 30 minutes and then list your name and the date on the line at the bottom of the last page. Please switch to a pen or pencil that writes in a different color after 15 minutes.

Wudzit Taique, a 47 year old Latvian woman recently provisionally

diagnosed with Dementia of the Alzheimer's Type (DAT) was referred by

Dr. Edward S. Hands, M.D. for this 01/01/2011 neuropychological evaluation.

Prior to her symptom onset, Ms. Taique reported being extremely active (i.e.

liked to paint, make stained glass, and attending the opera) but she tearfully

related that she is no longer interested in these hobbies. Her recent activities have consisted only of sipping vodka and watching Fox News.

Her husband, a long-haul tractor-trailer driver and stamp collector, reports

observing cognitive symptoms in his wife for the past six months. He also said

she will emit gasping and snorting sounds when she sleeps.

They live locally with there preschool-age grandchild, who they adopted

following the death of the child's parents last year.

Ms. Taique immigrated from Latvia two years ago. She completed 12 years

of schooling in Russian and Mining Technology. She then worked as a coal minor

for several years until developing chronic back pain from a 1975 mining accident.

Currently prescribed medications consist of Oxycontin, Nardil, and

Hydrocodone, and she discontinued Luvox two days ago due to side affects.

She also takes about two asprin every four to six hours.

Ms. Taique's vision was determined to be adequate to participate in testing, as was her hearing, despite her complaint of tinnitis. Test results are considered

a valid reflection of her current cognitive ability.

Her Full Scale IQ is 112 (VCI = 107; PRI = 103; WMI = 104; PSI = 105).

Thus, Ms. Taique's current overall intellectual functioning tested as superior, with

verbal abilities significantly stronger than nonverbal abilities. She demonstrated

relative strength in arithmetic, as indicated by her Digit Span scaled score of 12,

which falls at the 84th%ile. On the Trail Making Test, Mr. Taique scored in the

mild-deficit range (32nd%ile) compared to others her age group, however, this

measure is not particularly sensitive to neurologic dysfunction. Language abilities

appeared intact, as performance on multiple measures of reading, spelling, compre-hension, design fluency, and word-finding abilities were normal. Memory

testing revealed deficits in list learning and free recall, while recognition tested as normal, suggesting problems involving both retention and retrieval.

Ms. Taique scored in the normal range (T=67) on Scale 7 of the MMPI-2,

and there are no other indications of depression.

In conclusion, assessment results are consistent with a diagnosis of DAT.

Pre- and Post-Test Scoring

A scoring key is provided as an appendix so that you can see how much you learned by reviewing these guidelines.

Assign 1 point for each <u>knowledge</u> (K), <u>writing ability</u> (W), and <u>common sense</u> (C) correction and 6 points for each <u>follow-through</u> (F) task completed, for a maximum score of 80.

For those who are curious about how others do, a score of 28/80 on the pre-test falls at the approximate mean for applicants to our training program, while a score of 38/80 falls about one standard deviation above the mean. Keep in mind, though, that this is just a training exercise and not a formally developed psychological test.

Part II
Formats: Questionnaires and Reports

Most neuropsychologists eventually develop their own formats or templates to speed up the process of report writing. Ideally, these tools provide enough structure to promote efficiency, but not so much that reports have a "cookie-cutter" or fill-in-the-blank appearance. Two examples of report templates are provided, one more suited for medical settings, where brevity is appreciated, and one more suited for forensic settings, where thoroughness is expected.

To further facilitate report preparation, it helps to have questionnaires structured to gather background information in the same order that it will be presented in the report. Two such questionnaires are provided, one for patients capable of filling out their own and one for family members to fill out.

Purchasers of this book are free to modify report formats and questionnaires for use in their own practices and may request editable versions from the author by contacting NeuRules@gmail.com.

The first questionnaire presented below is for patients to fill out themselves, ideally prior to the interview. Additional notes can be made by the examiner on the questionnaire during the interview so that background information is organized and ready to insert into the report. Use of a different color of ink when making such notes is helpful in case questions ever arise in a deposition about who wrote what information.

A family report version of this questionnaire is also provided.

Chapter 11
Self-Report Questionnaire

Most of this questionnaire is self-explanatory, but there are two pages that require some explanation.

The two pages that begin with "**Step 1**" are designed to elicit reports about depression and anxiety symptoms both before and after the relevant injury or illness. Please note that on both pages items 16-19 are designed to alert the examiner to the possibility that formal assessment for validity of psychological symptom reporting may be useful. (The even items may reflect over-reporting, while the odd items may reflect under-reporting, and the pre/post comparison may also be revealing.)

R.L. Wanlass, *The Neuropsychology Toolkit: Guidelines, Formats, and Language*,
DOI 10.1007/ 978-1-4614-1882-5_11, © Springer Science+Business Media, LLC 2012

Neuropsychological Questionnaire

Self-Report Version

Please answer these questions to the best of your ability and bring this form to your appointment with Dr. _____ **on** _____
at _____.

IDENTIFYING INFORMATION:

Name   : _____

Date of Birth : _____

Age   : _____

Phone #   : _____

Address   : _____

_____

REFERRAL INFORMATION:

Who referred you for this evaluation? _____

_____

What information would you like to gain through this evaluation? _____

_____

_____

HISTORY OF CURRENT PROBLEM/INJURY/ILLNESS:

1. **Date** injury or illness started: _____/_____/_____

2. Illness/injury can be labeled as:

   _____ Head injury

   _____ Stroke

   _____ Other (please specify): _____

3. Please describe in detail the **accident or illness**: _____

   _____

   _____

   _____

_____

_____

_____

_____

_____

_____

_____

_____

_____

_____

4. Were you taken to an **emergency room**? __Yes, __ No. If yes, where? _____

_____

5. Were you **hospitalized**? __Yes, __No. If yes, where? _____

_____

6. What **diagnostic** procedures (e.g., **CT** scan, **MRI** scan, **EEG**) have been done and what were the results? _____

_____

7. Did you have **surgery**? __ Yes, __ No. If yes, for what? _____

_____

_____

8. Were there any **complications** such as increased intracranial (in the head) pressure/swelling, meningitis or infection? __ Yes, __ No. If yes, please describe: _____

_____

9. Did you receive **inpatient** rehabilitation services? __Yes, __No. If yes, please describe: _____

_____

10. Did you receive **outpatient** rehabilitation services? __Yes, __No. If yes, please describe: _____

_____

_____

11. Do you **still** have any **pain** or other **physical problems**? __Yes, __No. If yes, please describe: _____

_____

_____

_____

_____

_____

_____

12. Please list any medications you **currently** take:

Medication	**Dosage**
1. _____	_____
2. _____	_____
3. _____	_____
4. _____	_____
5. _____	_____

13. Please describe **current alcohol** use in terms of what you drink, how much, and how often: _____

14. Please describe **current street drug** use in terms of what you use, how much and how often: _____

_____

15. Please describe any **current** exposure to **toxic substances** (e.g., solvents, pesticides, lead) in your workplace or living environment: _____

PRIOR MEDICAL HISTORY:

1. Were you born: ____ on time, ____ prematurely, or ____ late?

2. What was your **birth weight**? ____ lbs., ____ oz.

3. Please describe any problems you are aware of that were associated with your birth or the immediate time period after birth: ___ oxygen deprivation, ___ unusual birth position, _____other (please describe): _____

_____

4. Please check all that applied to your mother while she was **pregnant** with you:

____ Alcohol use ____Cigarette smoking

____ Recreational or street drug use ____ Malnutrition

____ Exposure to environmental toxins ____ Accidents

5. List all medications (prescribed or over-the-counter) your mother took while pregnant: _____

_____

6. Did your **developmental progress**, such as walking and talking, occur ＿＿＿ early, ＿＿＿ average, or ＿＿＿ late?

7. As a child, did you have any developmental problems? If so, please describe:
＿＿＿＿＿＿＿＿＿＿＿＿＿＿＿＿＿＿＿＿＿＿＿＿＿＿＿＿＿＿＿＿＿＿＿

8. As a child, were you around any toxic waste, toxic fumes of any kind, or lead? ＿＿＿ Yes / ＿＿＿ No. If yes, please explain: ＿＿＿＿＿＿＿＿＿＿＿＿＿＿＿

9. How was your **nutrition** in childhood? ＿＿＿＿＿＿＿＿＿＿＿＿＿＿＿＿＿

10. Please describe any psychiatric, neurological (including dementia), substance abuse, or academic problems that **close relatives** have had: ＿＿＿＿＿＿＿＿
＿＿＿＿＿＿＿＿＿＿＿＿＿＿＿＿＿＿＿＿＿＿＿＿＿＿＿＿＿＿＿＿＿＿＿

11. By whom were you raised? ＿＿＿＿＿＿＿＿＿＿＿＿＿＿＿＿＿＿＿＿＿＿＿

12. Please describe any **previous** concussion/loss of consciousness or other brain injury: ＿＿＿＿＿＿＿＿＿＿＿＿＿＿＿＿＿＿＿＿＿＿＿＿＿＿＿＿＿＿
＿＿＿＿＿＿＿＿＿＿＿＿＿＿＿＿＿＿＿＿＿＿＿＿＿＿＿＿＿＿＿＿＿＿＿

13. Please describe any **previous** hospitalization, neurological illness, serious injury, or surgery: ＿＿＿＿＿＿＿＿＿＿＿＿＿＿＿＿＿＿＿＿＿＿＿＿＿
＿＿＿＿＿＿＿＿＿＿＿＿＿＿＿＿＿＿＿＿＿＿＿＿＿＿＿＿＿＿＿＿＿＿＿
＿＿＿＿＿＿＿＿＿＿＿＿＿＿＿＿＿＿＿＿＿＿＿＿＿＿＿＿＿＿＿＿＿＿＿

14. Please list any other illnesses or health problems you have ever had: ＿＿＿＿＿
＿＿＿＿＿＿＿＿＿＿＿＿＿＿＿＿＿＿＿＿＿＿＿＿＿＿＿＿＿＿＿＿＿＿＿

15. Please describe any **history** of heavy or frequent **alcohol** use: ＿＿＿＿＿＿
＿＿＿＿＿＿＿＿＿＿＿＿＿＿＿＿＿＿＿＿＿＿＿＿＿＿＿＿＿＿＿＿＿＿＿

16. Please describe any **history** of heavy or frequent **drug** use: ＿＿＿＿＿＿＿
＿＿＿＿＿＿＿＿＿＿＿＿＿＿＿＿＿＿＿＿＿＿＿＿＿＿＿＿＿＿＿＿＿＿＿

17. Please describe any history of **legal or job problems** due to alcohol or drug use:＿＿＿＿＿＿＿＿＿＿＿＿＿＿＿＿＿＿＿＿＿＿＿＿＿＿＿＿＿＿＿
＿＿＿＿＿＿＿＿＿＿＿＿＿＿＿＿＿＿＿＿＿＿＿＿＿＿＿＿＿＿＿＿＿＿＿

18. Please describe any history of exposure to **environmental toxins** at work or elsewhere: ＿＿＿＿＿＿＿＿＿＿＿＿＿＿＿＿＿＿＿＿＿＿＿＿＿＿＿＿＿

19. Please describe any **mental health problems or diagnoses** you have ever had:
＿＿＿＿＿＿＿＿＿＿＿＿＿＿＿＿＿＿＿＿＿＿＿＿＿＿＿＿＿＿＿＿＿＿＿
＿＿＿＿＿＿＿＿＿＿＿＿＿＿＿＿＿＿＿＿＿＿＿＿＿＿＿＿＿＿＿＿＿＿＿

20. Please describe any **mental health treatment** you have ever received: ＿＿＿＿＿
＿＿＿＿＿＿＿＿＿＿＿＿＿＿＿＿＿＿＿＿＿＿＿＿＿＿＿＿＿＿＿＿＿＿＿
＿＿＿＿＿＿＿＿＿＿＿＿＿＿＿＿＿＿＿＿＿＿＿＿＿＿＿＿＿＿＿＿＿＿＿
＿＿＿＿＿＿＿＿＿＿＿＿＿＿＿＿＿＿＿＿＿＿＿＿＿＿＿＿＿＿＿＿＿＿＿

EDUCATIONAL AND CULTURAL BACKGROUND:

1. What is your **primary language**?: _____

2. What is your **cultural or ethnic background**?: _____

3. What is the **highest** grade that you completed in school? _____

4. Were you labeled as "**learning disabled**" or placed in any **special education** classes? ___ Yes, ___ No. If yes, please describe: _____
    _____
    _____

5. Did you have any **behavioral or disciplinary problems** in school? ___ Yes, ___No. If yes, please describe: _____
    _____
    _____

6. Did you **repeat any grades**? __ Yes, __No. If yes, please describe: _____
    _____

7. What were your **best subjects**? _____
    _____

8. What were your **worst subjects**? _____
    _____

9. As a student, were you _____ average, _____ above average, or _____ below average?

10. Please describe any **grade point averages** or **standardized test scores** (e.g., SAT, IQ, achievement tests, etc.) that you earned: _____
    _____
    _____
    _____

11. Please describe any **special accomplishments or strengths** as a student: _____
    _____
    _____

WORK HISTORY:

1. Were you ever in the **military**? __ Yes, __No. If yes, what rank and branch? ___
   _____ For how long? _____ Type of discharge: _____
   Military jobs included: _____

2. **Prior jobs** (please **start with the most recent**):
   Months/Years

   a. _____
   b. _____
   c. _____
   d. _____
   e. _____

3. What work were you doing **at the time of your injury/illness**? _____
   _____
   For how long? _____ Salary? _____

4. Did you continue to work at this job after your injury/illness? _____ Yes, ___ No

5. What is your **current job**, if any? _____

CURRENT LIVING SITUATION:

1. Currently, are you married, divorced, separated, single? _____

2. Who lives with you? _____

3. Where do you live?_____

4. Is anyone your **conservator or legal guardian**?_____

5. Please describe your **typical daily activities**: _____
   _____
   _____
   _____

6. What **help or supervision** do you need from others? _____
   _____
   _____

7. Do you currently drive? _____

8. Do you have a **valid** driver's license? _____

9. Do you currently have **seizures**? _____

10. Do you rely on your own car, a borrowed car, rides from friends or family, or public transportation? _____

11. What is your current source of income or financial support? _____
    _____

12. Have you been involved in **lawsuits** for this or any other injury?___ Yes, ___ No
    If yes, please describe the outcome or current status: _____

PROBLEMS:

Please describe the problems you are having **now** and indicate whether you **also** had these problems **before** your injury or illness.

	Now	**Before**

1. Difficulty with **problem solving or reasoning**? _____ _____
   If so, please describe: _____
   _____

2. Problems with **speed of thinking**? _____ _____
   If so, please describe: _____
   _____

3. Problems with **concentration**? _____ _____
   If so, please describe: _____
   _____

4. Problems with **memory**? _____ _____
   If so, please describe: _____
   _____

5. Problems with **speaking, listening, writing,** _____ _____
   or reading? If so, please describe: _____
   _____

6. Problems with **strength or coordination**? _____ _____
   If so, please describe: _____
   _____

7. Problems with **vision**? _____ _____
   If so, please describe: _____
   _____

8. Problems with **spatial** ability or sense of direction? _____ _____
   If so, please describe: _____
   _____

9. Problems with sense of **hearing, touch, or smell**? _____ _____
   If so, please describe: _____
   _____

10. Problems with **psychological or social adjustment**
    or aspects of your life that are **stressful**? _____ _____
    If so, please describe: _____
    _____

Step 1: Please read through each statement below and indicate how well each one describes how you have been over the past 2 weeks?

Step 2: Go back through each statement and indicate how you were right before your injury or illness.

	Over the Past Two Weeks:			Before my Injury or Illness:		
	False	Partly True	Very True	False	Partly True	Very True
1. I often feel sad or empty.						
2. I have lost interest in most things.						
3. I don't enjoy the things that I am able to do.						
4. I don't laugh or smile much any more.						
5. Things bother or annoy me more easily now.						
6. I often feel like crying.						
7. I don't care much about other people any more.						
8. I often feel like a failure.						
9. I feel very bad about things I have done						
10. I don't feel much romantic or physical attraction towards anyone.						
11. I don't have much that I want to do.						
12. I don't have much to look forward to.						
13. I often think about dying.						
14. My life does not seem worth much.						
15. I don't care much whether I live or die.						
16. I feel like the most unhappy person on earth.						
17. I never feel down or discouraged.						
18. I am depressed, and my mood stays the same all day long every day.						
19. My thoughts are always cheerful.						
20. I often feel restless.						
21. I often feel tired or slowed down.						
22. I sleep too much.						
23. It is hard for me to stay asleep.						
24. It is hard to think, concentrate, or make decisions.						
25. I eat too little or too much.						

Step 1: Please read through each statement below and indicate how well each one describes how you have been over the past 2 weeks?

Step 2: Go back through each statement and indicate how you were right before your injury or illness.

	Over the Past Two Weeks:			Before my Injury or Illness:		
	False	Partly True	Very True	False	Partly True	Very True
1. I seem to worry more than others.						
2. I lack confidence.						
3. I have so many worries that it is hard to relax.						
4. I rarely feel safe and secure.						
5. I feel a sense of fear or dread.						
6. I often have feelings of intense fear or panic when there is no real danger.						
7. I often have fears about going crazy.						
8. I have much stronger fears than most people about certain things, places, or activities.						
9. Because of fear, I avoid activities, things, or places that most people would not avoid.						
10. Bad memories or nightmares often bother me.						
11. I am more jumpy or easily startled than others.						
12. I often try to avoid certain social situations because they make me nervous.						
13. I often worry about what others think of me.						
14. Often I can't stop doing things over and over (like counting, re-checking, washing, or cleaning).						
15. Often I can't stop certain distressing thoughts from running through my mind.						
16. I have been too stressed to be able to sleep at all.						
17. I am always confident.						
18. I constantly feel startled.						
19. I have no fears or worries.						
20. I have fears that I am about to die or lose control.						
21. I worry so much that it is hard to fall asleep.						
22. My muscles are tense or tight from stress or worry.						
23. I often sweat from stress even when it's not hot.						
24. I am often so nervous that my breath or heart rate seems to speed up or become uneven.						

This form should be filled out by someone (e.g., co-worker, supervisor, friend, relative) who has known you well before and after your injury or illness.
Please describe the problems _____ is having **now** and indicate whether he/she **also** had these problems **before** the _____ injury/illness. Please put **your** name, relationship to the person you are describing, and today's date here: __

	Now	Before
1. Difficulty with **problem solving or reasoning**?	_____	_____
If so, please describe: _____		
2. Problems with **speed of thinking**?	_____	_____
If so, please describe: _____		
3. Problems with **concentration**?	_____	_____
If so, please describe: _____		
4. Problems with **memory**?	_____	_____
If so, please describe: _____		
5. Problems with **speaking, listening, writing, or reading**?	_____	_____
If so, please describe: _____		
6. Problems with **strength or coordination**?	_____	_____
If so, please describe: _____		
7. Problems with **vision**?	_____	_____
If so, please describe: _____		
8. Problems with **spatial** ability or sense of direction?	_____	_____
If so, please describe: _____		
9. Problems with sense of **hearing, touch, or smell**?	_____	_____
If so, please describe: _____		
10. Problems with **psychological or social adjustment** or aspects of his/her life that are **stressful**?	_____	_____
If so, please describe: _____		

Chapter 12
Family Report Questionnaire

This is a re-worded version of the self-report questionnaire for use in cases in which the patient lacks either the time or the ability to provide background information in writing. When corroboration or extra detail is important, this questionnaire may also be used to gather supplemental information even in cases in which the patient does complete the self-report version.

R.L. Wanlass, *The Neuropsychology Toolkit: Guidelines, Formats, and Language*,
DOI 10.1007/ 978-1-4614-1882-5_12, © Springer Science+Business Media, LLC 2012

Neuropsychological Questionnaire

Family Version (Completed by: _____)
Please answer to the best of your ability the following questions about:
_____

IDENTIFYING INFORMATION:

Name: _____

Date of Birth: _____

Age: _____

Phone #:   _____

Address: _____

                              _____

REFERRAL INFORMATION:

Who referred him/her for this evaluation? _____

What information would you and he/she like to gain through this evaluation? ____

_____

HISTORY OF CURRENT PROBLEM/ILLNESS:

1. **Date** injury or illness started: ___/___/___

2. Illness/injury can be labeled as:

    _____ Head injury

    _____ Stroke

    _____ Other (please specify): _____

3. Please describe in detail the **accident or illness**: _____

_____

_____

_____

_____

_____

_____

_____

_____

_____

_____

_____

_____

_____

4. Was he/she taken to an **emergency room**? __Yes, __ No. If yes, where? _____

_____

5. Was he/she **hospitalized**? __Yes, __No. If yes, where? _____

_____

6. What **diagnostic** procedures (e.g., **CT** scan, **MRI** scan, **EEG**) have been done and what were the results? _____

_____

7. Did he/she have **surgery**? __ Yes, __ No. If yes, for what? _____

_____

_____

8. Were there any **complications** such as increased intracranial (in the head) pressure/swelling, meningitis or infection? If so, please describe: _____

_____

9. Did he/she receive **inpatient** rehabilitation services? _Yes, __No. If yes, please describe: _____

_____

10. Did he/she receive **outpatient** rehabilitation services? __Yes, __No. If yes, please describe: _____

_____

_____

11 Does he/she **still** have any **pain** or other **physical problems**? ___Yes, ___No. If yes, please describe: _____

_____

_____

_____

_____

12. Please list any medications he/she **currently** takes:

            Medication   **Dosage**

    1. _____   _____

    2. _____   _____

    3. _____   _____

    4. _____   _____

    5. _____   _____

13. Please describe **current alcohol** use in terms of what, how much, and how often he/she drinks: _____
_____

14. Please describe current **street drug** use in terms of what he/she uses, how much and how often: _____

15. Please describe any **current** exposure to **toxic substances** (e.g., solvents, pesticides, lead) in his/her workplace or living environment: _____
_____

PRIOR MEDICAL HISTORY:

1. Was he/she born: _____ on time, _____ prematurely, or _____ late?

2. What was his/her **birth weight**? _____ lbs., _____ oz.

3. Please describe any problems you are aware of that were associated with birth or the immediate time period after birth: _____ oxygen deprivation, _____ unusual birth position, other (please describe): _____

4. Please check all that applied to his/her mother while she was **pregnant** with him/her:
   _____ Alcohol use _____ Cigarette smoking

   _____ Recreational or street drug use _____ Malnutrition

   _____ Exposure to environmental toxins _____ Accidents

5. List all medications (prescribed or over-the-counter) his/her mother took while pregnant: _____

6. Did his/her **developmental progress**, such as walking and talking, occur _____ early, _____ average, or _____ late?

7. As a child, did he/she have any developmental problems? If so, please describe:
_____

8. As a child, was he/she around any toxic waste, toxic fumes of any kind, or lead? ___ Yes / ___ No. If yes, please explain: _____

9. How was his/her **nutrition** in childhood? _____

10. Please describe any psychiatric, neurological (including dementia), substance abuse, or academic problems that **close relatives** have had: _____
_____

11. By whom was he/she raised? _____

12. Please describe any **previous** concussion/loss of consciousness or other brain injury: _____
_____
_____

13. Please describe any **previous** hospitalization, neurologic illness, serious injury, or surgery: _____
_____

14. Please list any other illnesses or health problems he/she has ever had: _____
_____

15. Please describe any **history** of heavy or frequent **alcohol** use: _____
_____
_____

16. Please describe any **history** of heavy or frequent **drug** use: _____
_____
_____

17. Please describe any history of **legal or job problems** due to alcohol or drugs:
_____

18. Please describe any history of exposure to **environmental toxins** at work or elsewhere: _____

19. Please describe any **mental health problems or diagnoses** he/she has ever had: _____

20. Please describe any **mental health treatment** he/she has ever received: _____
_____
_____

EDUCATIONAL AND CULTURAL BACKGROUND:

1. What is his/her **primary language**?: _____

2. What is his/her **cultural or ethnic background**?: _____

3. What is the **highest** grade that he/she completed in school? _____

4. Was he/she labeled as "**learning disabled**" or placed in any **special education** classes? ____ Yes, ____ No. If yes, please describe: _____
   _____
   _____

5. Did he/she have any **behavioral or disciplinary problems** in school?
   __ Yes, __No. If yes, please describe: _____
   _____
   _____

6. Did he/she **repeat any grades**? __ Yes, __No. If yes, please describe: _____
   _____

7. What were his/her **best subjects**? _____

8. What were his/her **worst subjects**? _____

9. As a student, was he/she
   _____ average, _____ above average, or _____ below average?

10. Please describe any **grade point averages** or **standardized test scores** (e.g., SAT, IQ, achievement tests, etc.) that he/she earned: _____
    _____
    _____
    _____
    _____

11. Please describe any **special accomplishments or strengths** as a student: ____
    _____

WORK HISTORY:

1. Was he/she ever in the **military**? __ Yes, __No.
   If yes, what rank and branch? _____ For how long? _____
   Type of discharge: _____ Military jobs included: _____

2. **Prior jobs** (please **start with the most recent**): **Months/Years**
   a. _____
   b. _____
   c. _____
   d. _____
   e. _____
   f. _____
   g. _____

3. What work was he/she doing **at the time of his/her injury/illness**? _____
   _____
   _____

   For how long? _____ Salary? _____
   Did he/she continue to work at this job after his/her injury/illness? __ Yes, __ No

4. What is his/her **current job**, if any? _____
   _____
   _____
   _____

CURRENT LIVING SITUATION:

1. Currently, is he/she married, divorced, separated, single? _____

2. Who lives with him/her? _____

3. Where does he/she live? _____

4. Is anyone his/her **conservator or legal guardian**? _____

5. Please describe his/her **typical daily activities**: _____
   _____
   _____
   _____
   _____
   _____
   _____
   _____

6. What **help or supervision** does he/she need from others? _____

_____

_____

_____

_____

_____

7. Does he/she currently drive? _____

8. Does he/she have a **valid** driver's license? _____

9. Does he/she currently have **seizures**? _____

10. Does he/she rely on his/her own car, a borrowed car, rides from friends or family, or public transportation? _____

11. What is his/her current source of income or financial support? _____

_____

_____

12. Has he/she been involved in **lawsuits** for this or any other injury? __ Yes, __ No

    If yes, please describe the outcome or current status: _____

_____

_____

PROBLEMS:

Please describe the problems he/she is having now and indicate whether he/she had these problems before his/her injury or illness.

	Now	Before

1. Difficulty with **problem solving or reasoning**? _____ _____

   If so, please describe: _____

   _____

2. Problems with **speed of thinking**? _____ _____

   If so, please describe: _____

   _____

3. Problems with **concentration**? _____ _____

   If so, please describe: _____

   _____

4. Problems with **memory**? _____ _____

   If so, please describe: _____

   _____

5. Problems with **speaking, listening, writing, or reading**? _____ _____

   If so, please describe: _____

   _____

6. Problems with **strength or coordination**? _____ _____

   If so, please describe: _____

   _____

7. Problems with **vision**? _____ _____

   If so, please describe: _____

   _____

8. Problems with **spatial** ability or sense of direction? _____ _____

   If so, please describe: _____

   _____

9. Problems with sense of **hearing, touch, or smell**? _____ _____

   If so, please describe: _____

   _____

10. Problems with **psychological or social adjustment** or aspects of his/her life that are **stressful**? _____ _____

    If so, please describe: _____

    _____

Chapter 13
Short Report Format

This brief report template is especially well suited for use in non-forensic medical settings or other contexts in which conciseness and rapid turn-around time are critical.

It will, of course, require some modification to suit the test battery preferences of each practitioner.

R.L. Wanlass, *The Neuropsychology Toolkit: Guidelines, Formats, and Language*,
DOI 10.1007/ 978-1-4614-1882-5_13, © Springer Science+Business Media, LLC 2012

NEUROPSYCHOLOGICAL EVALUATION

REFERRAL INFORMATION

Patient:	#:	DOB:	Age:

Referring Provider:

Reason for Referral: @ was referred for comprehensive assessment of cognitive and emotional functioning to provide treatment planning guidance for medical and other rehabilitation providers.

Location of Testing:

Date(s) of Evaluation:

HISTORY of CURRENT CONDITION

Date/Circumstances of Onset and Medical Diagnosis:

Rehabilitation Services:

Current Treatment/Medications:

Current Substance Use:

BACKGROUND INFORMATION

Developmental History:

Relevant Family Medical History:

Other Medical History:

Past Problematic Substance Use:

Psychiatric History:

Cultural/Linguistic Background:

Educational Background:

Grades/Standardized Test Performance:

Employment History:

Marital Status/Current Living Situation:

Typical Daily Activities:

Need for Supervision or Assistance:

Source of Income:

Driving Status:

TIME REQUIRED

Total Time Required =

SYSTEM for CATEGORIZING SCORES								
Severe Deficit: 3 SD or more below the mean	**Moderate Deficit**: 2 SD or more below the mean	**Mild Deficit**: 1 SD or more below the mean	**Low Average**: 2/3 SD or more below the mean	**Average**: >2/3 SD below the mean and <2/3 SD above the mean	**High Average**: 2/3 SD or more above the mean	**Superior**: 1 SD or more above the mean	**Very Superior**: 2 SD or more above the mean	**Exceptional**: 3 SD or more above the mean

Scores ranging from low average through high average are considered to be within normal limits (**WNL**). When appropriate and to the extent possible, norms have been selected to take the subject's demographic factors, such as age, gender, and education, into account.

COGNITIVE ASSESSMENT RESULTS			
FACTORS INFLUENCING TEST VALIDITY			
Function	*Test*	*Performance Level*	*Raw Score*
Effort	TOMM I		
	TOMM II		
	TOMM Retention		
	MSVT IR		
	MSVT DR		
	MSVT C		
	MSVT PA		
	MSVT FR		
	RFIT		
	RFIT Recall + Recognition		
Current Pain Self-Rating:			
Other Potential Test Confounds:			
Summary of Test Validity:			

INTELLECTUAL and PROBLEM-SOLVING ABILITY					
Problems Reported:					
Function	*Test*	*Performance Level*	*%ile*	*Standard Score*	*Raw Score*
Overall Intelligence	WAIS-IV Full Scale IQ			FSIQ =	sss =
Verbal Reasoning	WAIS-IV Verbal Comprehension Index			VCI =	sss =
Nonverbal Reasoning	WAIS-IV Perceptual Reasoning Index			PRI =	sss =
Abstract Verbal Reasoning	WAIS-IV Similarities			ss =	/36
Abstract Nonverbal Reasoning	WAIS-IV Matrix Reasoning			ss =	/26

INTELLECTUAL and PROBLEM-SOLVING ABILITY					
Problems Reported:					
Function	*Test*	*Performance Level*	*%ile*	*Standard Score*	*Raw Score*
Mental Arithmetic Reasoning	WAIS-IV Arithmetic			ss =	/22
Written Arithmetic Calculation	WRAT-4 Arithmetic				/55
Safety Judgment	NAB			T =	/20
	Independent Living Scales (ILS)			T =	/40
Money Management	Independent Living Scales			T =	/34
Managing Home and Transportation	Independent Living Scales			T =	/30
Adaptive Reasoning	Category Test			T =	/208 errors
Premorbid Intellectual Ability Estimate	Test of Premorbid Functioning (TOPF): Word Reading Predicted IQ			Est. FSIQ =	/70
	TOPF: Demographic Predicted IQ			Est. FSIQ =	
Summary of Intellectual and Problem-Solving Functions:					

PROCESSING SPEED					
Problems Reported:					
Observations:					
Function	*Test*	*Performance Level*	*%ile*	*Standard Score*	*Raw Score*
Psychomotor Speed	WAIS-IV PSI			PSI =	sss =
	WAIS-IV Digit Symbol-Coding			ss =	/135
	WAIS-IV Symbol Search			ss =	/60
	Digit Vigilance Test-Time			T =	''
	Trail Making Test, Part-A			T =	''
Verbal Fluency	COWAT (FAS)			T =	
	Animal Naming			T =	
Summary of Processing Speed:					

MENTAL CONTROL					
Problems Reported:					
Observations:					
Function	*Test*	*Performance Level*	*%ile*	*Standard Score*	*Raw Score*
Auditory Attention Span	WAIS-IV Digit Span (forward digit recall)			ss =	
Working Memory	WAIS-IV WMI			WMI =	sss =
	WAIS-IV Digit Span (backward digit recall)			ss =	
	WAIS-IV Digit Span Sequencing			ss =	
Mental Flexibility	Trail Making Test, Part-B			T =	"
	D-KEFS Color-Word Interference: Inhibition/ Switching			ss =	"
				ss =	errors
Selective Attention	D-KEFS Color-Word Interference: Inhibition			ss =	"
				ss =	errors
Sustained Visual Attention	Digit Vigilance Test- Errors				errors
Summary of Mental Control:					

LEARNING and MEMORY					
Problems Reported:					
Observations:					
Function	*Test*	*Performance Level*	*%ile*	*Standard Score*	*Raw Score*
Orientation	Cognistat Orientation				/12
Remote Memory/ Fund of Knowledge	WAIS-IV Information			ss =	/26
Verbal Learning & Memory					
Word List Learning	Rey Auditory Verbal Learning Test (RAVLT)			z =	/75
Post-Distraction Recall				z =	/15
Delayed Free Recall				z =	/15
List Recognition				z =	/15 *** FP
Story Recall- Immediate	WMS-IV Logical Memory			ss =	
Story Recall- 30-Minute Delay				ss =	

Visual Learning & Memory					
Design Recall- 3-Minute Delay	Rey Complex Figure Test			T =	/36
Design Recall- 30-Minute Delay				T =	/36
Design Recognition				T =	/24
Summary of Learning and Memory Functions:					

COMMUNICATION						
Problems Reported:						
Observations:						
Function	*Test*	*Performance Level*	*%ile*	*Standard Score*	*Raw Score*	
Listening Comprehension	Complex Ideational Material Test			T =	/12	
	Cognistat Comprehension				/6	
Naming/Word Finding	Boston Naming Test			T =	/60	
Repetition	Cognistat Repetition				/12	
Spelling	WRAT-4				/57	
Word Reading					/70	
Sentence Comprehension					/50	
Vocabulary	WAIS-IV Vocabulary			ss =	/57	
Summary of Communication Functions:						

MOTOR FUNCTIONS						
Problems Reported:						
Handedness:	Ambulation:					
Other Observations:						
Function	*Test*	*Performance Level*	*%ile*	*Standard Score*	*Raw Score*	
Manual Dexterity	Grooved Pegboard- Dominant Hand			T =	"	
	Grooved Pegboard- Nondominant Hand			T =	"	
Motor Speed	Finger Oscillation- Dominant Hand			T =		
	Finger Oscillation— Nondominant Hand			T =		
Grip Strength	Hand Dynamometer- Dominant Hand			T =	kg	
	Hand Dynamometer- Nondominant Hand			T =	kg	
Summary of Motor Functions:						

VISUAL-SPATIAL FUNCTIONS					
Problems Reported:					
Corrective Lenses Used for Testing?:					
Evidence of Visual Neglect:			Evidence of Right-Left Disorientation:		
Other Observations:					
Function	*Test*	*Performance Level*	*%ile*	*Standard Score*	*Raw Score*
Near Vision Acuity	Vision Screen	**20/**			
Color Vision					
Sustained Visual Attention	Digit Vigilance Test-Errors			T =	errors
Visual Processing/ Spatial Relations	WAIS-IV Visual Puzzles			ss =	/26
Scanning Efficiency	Trail Making Test, Part A			T =	"
Block Construction	WAIS-IV Block Design			ss =	/66
Figure Copy	Rey Complex Figure Test			z =	/36
Summary of Visual-Spatial Functions:					

MENTAL STATUS and PSYCHOLOGICAL ADJUSTMENT
Presentation and Appearance:
Affect Range and Appropriateness:

Evidence of Depressed Mood: On the Hospital Anxiety and Depression Scale (HADS), @ obtained a Depression raw score of ***/21, which falls in the *** range.

On the Symptom Checklist-90-R (SCL-90-R) Depression Scale, @ obtained a T-score of ***, which falls in the *** range.

@'s degree of endorsement of symptoms that can be indicative of depression is indicated below:

++ = Very True   **+ = Partly True**   **Empty = False**

Sadness		Social detachment		Diminished hope		Fatigue/lethargy	
Loss of interest		Failure feelings		Thoughts of death		Excessive sleep	
Loss of enjoyment		Guilt		Reduced self-worth		Impaired sleep maintenance	
Loss of humor		Reduced libido		Diminished will to live		Perceived cognitive problems	
Irritability		Reduced motivation		Restlessness		Appetite changes	
Tearfulness							

Clinical interview revealed ***.

Evidence of Anxiety: On the HADS, @ obtained an Anxiety raw score of ***/21, which falls in the *** range.

On the Symptom Checklist-90-R (SCL-90-R) Anxiety Scale, @ obtained a T-score of ***, which also falls in the *** range.

@'s degree of endorsement of symptoms that can be indicative of anxiety is indicated below:

++ = **Very True**		+ = **Partly True**		**Empty = False**	
Worry		Fear of "going crazy"		Social avoidance		Initial insomnia	
Loss of confidence		Phobic fear		Self-consciousness		Muscle tension	
Difficulty relaxing		Phobic avoidance		Repetitive behavior		Perspiration	
Insecurity		Distressing memories/ nightmares		Repetitive thoughts		Breathing/heart rate change	
Dread		Heightened startle response		Fear of death/loss of control		Appetite/digestion change	
Panic							

Clinical interview revealed ***.

Current Life Stressors:

Evidence of Suicidal or Homicidal Ideation:

Behavioral Control:

Thought Process and Insight:

Summary of Mental Status and Psychological Adjustment:

SUMMARY and CONCLUSIONS

@ demonstrated ***.

Findings within specific domains of functioning are summarized below:
- Intellectual and Problem-Solving Functions:
- Processing Speed:
- Mental Control:
- Learning and Memory Functions:
- Communication Functions:
- Motor Functions:
- Visual-Spatial Functions:
- Mental Status and Psychological Adjustment:

DIAGNOSTIC IMPRESSION

Diagnostically, @'s present condition can be best characterized as:
- ***
- ***

RECOMMENDATIONS
•   ***
•   ***
•   ***
•   ***

Thank you for this interesting referral. If you have any questions or if I can be of further assistance, please call ***.

_____
***
***

Chapter 14
Long Report Format

This report format is more suited for medical-legal contexts such as workers' compensation, disability insurance, and personal injury. It prompts the writer to provide more extensive background information and provides for the reader a more comprehensive explanation of what has been assessed and why.

As with the short format, it will require some modification to suit the test battery preferences of each practitioner.

R.L. Wanlass, *The Neuropsychology Toolkit: Guidelines, Formats, and Language*,
DOI 10.1007/ 978-1-4614-1882-5_14, © Springer Science+Business Media, LLC 2012

NEUROPSYCHOLOGICAL EVALUATION

CONFIDENTIAL

Re   : _____

: _____

Date of Birth   : _____

Age   : _____

Date of Injury   : _____

Referral source   : _____

Insurer   : _____

Location of testing : _____

Date of evaluation : _____

Dear ***:

Thank you for this referral to determine @'s current level of neuropsychological functioning.

@ verbalized understanding of the purpose of this evaluation and the limitations in confidentiality inherent in this evaluation process. @ specifically consented for this report to be submitted to and possibly discussed with

@ expressed understanding that we were meeting only for the purpose of evaluation and not engaging in treatment or establishing an ongoing doctor-patient relationship.

This report is written as a professional-to-professional communication. Because of the sensitive nature of the material contained herein, it is recommended that this report not be released to @ without first allowing for explanation of these results by a professional experienced with providing neuropsychological testing feedback.

MEDICAL BACKGROUND

HISTORY OF CURRENT CONDITION

Self-Report

Description of Injury/Onset: @ stated that
Unconsciousness, Amnesia, or other Alteration in Consciousness: @ reported
Other Information:

Medical Record Review

Date	Source	Content

Emergency Assessment and Intervention: According to

Radiological and other Diagnostic Findings:

Surgical Procedures:

Rehabilitation Services:

Other Relevant Medical Information:

Current Physical Symptoms: When asked about current physical problems, @ reported

Current Medications:

Other Current Chemical Use or Exposure: When asked about current use of or exposure to alcohol, drugs, or toxins, @ reported

PRIOR MEDICAL HISTORY

Prenatal and Perinatal Factors: When asked about awareness of problems associated with gestation or delivery, @ reported

Early Development: The speed at which developmental milestones were reached was reported by @ to have been

Family History: @ was raised by

When questioned about awareness of family history of psychiatric, neurological, or academic problems, @ reported

Major Injuries

Prior Concussion, Loss of Consciousness, or Other Brain Injury: When questioned about any prior history of concussion, loss of consciousness, or other brain injury, @ reported

Other Serious Injury: In response to questioning about any other serious injury, @ responded

Major Illnesses or Surgeries

Neurological Illness or Surgery: When asked about any prior history of neurological illness or surgery, @ reported

Other Serious or Chronic Illness or Major Surgery: When questioned about any history of non-neurological illness or surgery, @

Chemical Exposure

History of Heavy or Frequent Alcohol Use: In response to a question about any history of heavy or frequent alcohol use, @ reported

History of Heavy or Frequent Drug Use: Regarding any history of heavy or frequent drug use, @ indicated

History of Legal or Occupational Problems Due to Substance Use: Previous legal or occupational problems associated with substance use were

History of Exposure to Occupational or Other Environmental Toxins: When questioned about any knowledge of prior exposure to occupational or other environmental toxins, @ indicated

Mental Health History

Problems/Diagnoses: In response to questioning about prior mental health problems or diagnoses, @ reported

Treatment: Prior mental health treatment has reportedly

SOCIAL BACKGROUND

EDUCATIONAL AND CULTURAL BACKGROUND

Language Background: @ reported a primary language of

Cultural/Ethnic Background: @'s self-described cultural/ethnic background is

Highest Level of Education: @ reported completing

Learning or Behavioral Problems: When asked about academic or behavioral problems in school, @ reported

Grades and/or Standardized Test Performance: Academic performance was reported by @ to have been

Special Accomplishments/Strengths: When asked about special accomplishments or strengths, @ reported

OCCUPATIONAL HISTORY

Military History: When questioned about history of military service, @ indicated

General Employment History Prior to Injury/Onset: @ reported a history of working

Employment at Time of Injury/Onset: @ was working

Employment Since Injury/Onset: @

CURRENT LIVING SITUATION

Place of Residence and Current Household Members: @ lives

Typical Daily Activities: When asked about current typical daily activities, @ replied

Need for Supervision or Assistance with Activities of Daily Living: In response to questioning about any need for supervision by others or assistance with activities of daily living, @ reported

Source of Income: @ reported current income from

EVALUATION PROCEDURES

RECORDS REVIEWED:

Neuropsychological Questionnaire completed by @
Neuropsychological Problem Inventory completed by informant:

CLINICAL INTERVIEW:

History and mental status interview with @

ASSESSMENT TOOLS UTILIZED:

Boston Naming Test (BNT)
Category Fluency (Animal Naming)
Category Test
Cognistat (Orientation, Repetition, Judgment, Comprehension)
Complex Ideational Material Test (CIMT)
Digit Vigilance Test (DVT)
Finger Tapping Test (FTT)
Grooved Pegboard Test (GPT)
Hand Dynamometer (HD)
Hospital Anxiety and Depression Scale (HADS)
Letter Fluency (FAS)
MSVT
Near Vision and Color Discrimination Screen
Paced Auditory Serial Addition Test (PASAT)
Personality Assessment Inventory (PAI)
Quick Smell Identification Test (QSIT)
RDS
Rey Auditory Verbal Learning Test (RAVLT)
Rey Fifteen-Item Test with Boone's Recognition (RFIT)
Rey-Osterreith Complex Figure Test (ROCFT)
Stroop Color-Word Test (Golden)
Symptom Checklist-90-Revised (SCL-90-R)
Test of Memory Malingering (TOMM)
Trail Making Test (TMT)
Wechsler Adult Intelligence Scale (WAIS-IV)
Wechsler Memory Scale-IV Logical Memory I and II
Wechsler Memory Scale-III Family Pictures I and II
Wechsler Test of Adult Reading (WTAR)
Wide Range Achievement Test (WRAT4)
WMT

SYSTEM FOR CATEGORIZING SCORES: On tests for which standardized scores (e.g., T-scores or percentiles) are available, a classification system is applied such that scores one standard deviation or more below the mean (less than or equal to the 16th percentile) are considered to fall in the *mild* deficit range. Scores two or more standard deviations below the mean (less than or equal to the 2nd percentile) are considered to fall in the *moderate* deficit range. Scores three or more standard deviations below the mean (less than or equal to the 0.1 percentile) are considered to fall in the *severe* deficit range.

Scores that are above the 16th percentile but not greater than the 25th percentile are designated as falling in the *low average* range. Scores falling above the 25th percentile and below the 75th percentile are classified as *average*. Scores ranging from the 75th percentile to just below the 84th percentile are categorized as *high average*. Scores within this broad band from just above the 16th percentile to just below the 84th percentile are considered *within normal limits*.

Scores falling far above average are labeled as *superior* (greater than or equal to the 84th percentile), *very superior* (greater than or equal to the 98th percentile), or *exceptional* (greater than or equal to the 99.9th percentile), depending upon whether they are one, two, or three standard deviations above the mean.

When appropriate and to the extent possible, norms are selected to take the subject's demographic factors, such as age and education, into account.

TIME REQUIRED FOR EVALUATION

Hours of clinical interview and face-to-face testing/evaluation:
Hours of test scoring, interpretation, and reporting:
Hours of record review:
Total hours required:

TEST VALIDITY ISSUES

POTENTIAL CONFOUNDS

Potential Linguistic or Cultural Confounds: Testing confounds related to @'s cultural and linguistic background were

Potential Emotional Confounds: Level of psychological distress was assessed in order to gauge whether any such distress was intense enough to be likely to significantly impede @'s ability to focus on test requirements. Based on this assessment,

Potential Medication/Other Substance Confounds: The possibility that medications or substances present in @'s system might affect test performance was considered. Problems of this type were

Potential Sensory or Motor Deficit Confounds: Careful attention was paid to make sure that @ could adequately see and hear stimuli and exercise adequate motor control to respond.

Potential Pain, Fatigue, or other Physical Condition Confounds: With 10 representing the worst imaginable pain and 0 representing no pain, @ reported a pain level of

Regarding fatigue or other physical condition confounds,

The influence of pain, fatigue, or other physical conditions on @'s ability to concentrate during testing was judged to be

Practice Effect from Prior Testing: Prior exposure to some of the same test materials

EFFORT/COOPERATION

Observed Effort: Effort exerted on testing appeared to be

Observed Consistency of Performance: Consistency of performance across similar tasks was judged to be

Results of Specific Testing of Effort/Cooperation: Prior to the initiation of testing, @ was advised of the importance of giving full effort. Performance on neuropsychological measures sensitive to effort and motivation suggests that cooperation was

TOMM raw score for Trial I =
TOMM raw score for Trial II =
TOMM raw score for Retention Trial =
RFIT raw score =
RFIT Recognition (free recall + {true positives-false positives}) =
RAVLT Recognition (Boone) =
RDS raw score =
WMT IR =
WMT DR =
WMT CNS =
WMT MC =
WMT PA =
WMT FR =
MSVT IR =
MSVT DR =
MSVT CNS =
MSVT PA =
MSVT FR =
PAI validity scales =
SCL-90-R PST raw score =

OVERALL ASSESSMENT OF TEST VALIDITY: The ability of testing to accurately reflect @'s current status is judged to be

NEUROPSYCHOLOGICAL FUNCTIONING

INTELLECTUAL AND PROBLEM-SOLVING ABILITY

Complaints

Self-Report:

Informant Report:

Test Findings

Intelligence Quotient: The IQ provides a useful summary score for various abilities that have been defined as constituting "intelligence," or the ability to reason, solve problems, think abstractly, plan, comprehend complex ideas, learn quickly, and learn from experience.

IQ tests do not assess all of the mental abilities necessary for successful functioning, which is why neuropsychological test batteries include many additional measures.

It is possible for a person with well-documented brain injury to obtain a normal-range IQ score if pre-injury intellectual ability was above normal or if the injury affected functions not well measured by the IQ test.

On current testing, @ obtained a Full Scale IQ score of

%ile for individuals in this age group =

Two major components of the Wechsler IQ test are the Verbal Comprehension Index (VCI), measuring verbal comprehension and reasoning ability, and the Perceptual Reasoning Index (PRI), measuring visual-perceptual organization and reasoning ability. Comparison of VCI to PRI reveals ***.

VCI =
%ile for individuals in this age group =

PRI =
%ile for individuals in this age group =

The General Ability Index (GAI) consists of the Similarities, Vocabulary, and Information subtests from the Verbal Comprehension Index and the Block Design, Matrix Reasoning, and Visual Puzzles subtests from the Perceptual Reasoning Index. The GAI, therefore, excludes measures of working memory and processing speed and consequently can be clinically useful as a measure of cognitive abilities that are less vulnerable to impairment.

GAI =
%ile for individuals in this age group =

Arithmetic Reasoning: Ability to mentally (i.e., with no paper or calculator) solve practical arithmetic problems tested in the

Test: Wechsler Arithmetic
Raw score =
Scaled score =
%ile for individuals in this age group =

Verbal Abstraction: On a verbal abstract reasoning task involving the identification of similarities between words, @ scored in the

Test: Wechsler Similarities
Raw score =
Scaled score =
%ile for individuals in this age group =

Nonverbal Reasoning: Ability to solve nonverbal reasoning problems tested in the

Test: Wechsler Matrix Reasoning
Raw score =
Scaled score =
%ile for individuals in this age group =

Adaptive Reasoning and Problem Solving: The Category Test has proven to be highly sensitive, often more so than IQ tests, to the reasoning and problem solving deficits that occur after brain injury. This test requires the ability to generate potential solutions to problems, test these in a systematic fashion (keeping track of which strategies work and which do not), and adapt flexibly as aspects of the problem change. @ obtained a Category Test score that falls in the

Errors on the Category Test =
%ile based on Heaton's demographically corrected norms =

Estimated Premorbid Intelligence

Premorbid Test Data: Records of premorbid cognitive testing were

Premorbid Academic and Vocational Attainment: @'s level of academic and vocational attainment suggests premorbid functioning in the

Estimate Based on Reading Ability and Demographics: Performance on word recognition/pronunciation tasks is generally more resistant to decline in the presence of brain impairment than most other cognitive functions and is sometimes used as an indication of premorbid intellectual status. (Such predictions can, however, overestimate the IQ of persons of very low intelligence and underestimate the IQ of persons of very high intelligence. Also, the presence of a reading disability obviously reduces the validity of this prediction method.) Using this method, premorbid Full Scale IQ is estimated to have been approximately

When demographic factors, such as level of education, are combined into the prediction equation along with the reading score, @'s premorbid Full Scale IQ is estimated to have been approximately

Test: Wechsler Test of Adult Reading (WTAR)
Raw score =

"Hold" Tests: Certain test scores (e.g., Picture Completion, Information) are less likely to show decline in the presence of most types of neurological insult and are therefore viewed as providing information about premorbid status. Results from "hold" tests suggest that premorbid ability was

Conclusions Regarding Premorbid Intelligence: @'s premorbid intellectual ability is estimated to have been

Conclusions Regarding Intellectual and Problem-Solving Ability:

PROCESSING SPEED

Complaints

Self-Report:

Informant Report:

Observational Data: Mental speed exhibited during several hours of interaction appeared

Test Findings

Processing Speed on Visual-Motor Tasks: Processing speed can be inferred by rate of completion on a digit-symbol substitution (or "coding") task in which the subject refers to a legend or key to translate numbers into their corresponding symbols. On this task, @ scored in the

Test: Wechsler Coding
Raw score =
Scaled score =
%ile for individuals in this age group =

Processing speed can also be inferred from the rate of completion on a visual search task requiring the subject to scan lines as rapidly as possible to detect the presence of matching symbols. On this task, @ scored in the

Test: Wechsler Symbol Search
Raw score =
Scaled score =
%ile for individuals in this age group =

Wechsler combines scores on the Coding and Symbol Search tasks into a composite score called the Processing Speed Index (PSI). On this index, @ scored in the

PSI standard score =
%ile for individuals in this age group =

On a task requiring the subject to rapidly search for target symbols among distracting symbols, @ performed in the

Test: DVT
Raw score in seconds =
%ile based on Heaton's demographically corrected norms =

Part A of the Trail Making Test (TMT-A) is a connect-the-dot task that requires rapid location of targets on a page, and time taken to complete this task can be used to draw inferences about visual scanning speed. @ performed in the

Seconds to complete this task =
%ile based on Heaton's demographically corrected norms =

Processing Speed on Tasks Requiring Spoken Output: On a task requiring the rapid reading of common words (i.e., color names), @ tested in the

Words read in 45 seconds =
%ile based on age- and education-corrected norms =

On a task requiring the rapid identification of colors, @ tested in the

Colors identified in 45 seconds =
%ile based on age- and education-corrected norms =

Verbal fluency refers to the ability to generate as many words as possible beginning with a specific letter or falling within a specific category while working under a time limit. This task requires speed in generating new words, preferably utilizing working memory to avoid repetition of words. @ performed in the

Test: Animal Naming
Raw score =
%ile based on Heaton's demographically corrected norms =

Test: FAS
Raw score =
%ile based on Heaton's demographically corrected norms =

Test: Thurstone
Raw score =
%ile based on Heaton's demographically corrected norms =

Conclusions Regarding Processing Speed: Analysis of scores on tests of mental speed indicates

MENTAL CONTROL

Complaints

Self-Report:

Informant Report:

Test Findings

Auditory Attention Span: The forward digit recall task is a measure of attention and concentration. The subject is required to listen carefully to a series of numbers. Then, the subject is to repeat that string of numbers in the same order. @ scored in the

Maximum digits recalled in the forward direction =
Raw score for digits forward =
%ile for individuals in this age group =

Working Memory: Working memory can be defined simply as the memory that holds information we are using at the time.

One measure of working memory is backward digit recall, which requires the ability to hold information (i.e., a series of numbers) in temporary storage while performing a mental manipulation (i.e., reversal) on it. On the Wechsler digits reverse task, @ scored in the

Maximum digits recalled in the reverse direction =
Raw score for digits reverse =
%ile for individuals in this age group =

The Wechsler Digit Span subtest includes recall of digit sequences in the forward and backward directions, as well as recall of randomly presented digits after mentally rearranging them into numerical order. On this Digit Span task, @ scored in the ***.

Raw score for Digit Span (digits forward + reverse) =
Scaled score =
%ile for individuals in this age group =

Wechsler's Letter-Number Sequencing (LNS) task requires the examinee to hold a series of randomly ordered letters and numbers in working memory long enough to reorganize them into proper sequence. On this task, @ scored in the

Raw score for Letter-Number Sequencing =
Scaled score =
%ile for individuals in this age group =

Wechsler combines scores on the Digit Span and Arithmetic subtests into a composite score called the Working Memory Index (WMI). On this index, @ scored in the

WMI standard score =
%ile for individuals in this age group =

The Paced Auditory Serial Addition Test (PASAT) requires ability to hold numbers in working memory while rapidly performing simple mental arithmetic as the speed requirement increases across trials. @ obtained a total score that falls in the

Series 1 correct =
Series 2 correct =
Series 3 correct =
Series 4 correct =
Total correct =
%ile based on Heaton's demographically corrected norms =

Mental Flexibility/Alternating Attention: Trail Making Test Part B (TMT-B) is a connect-the-dot task that requires the subject to alternate between consecutive numbers and letters as rapidly as possible. On this task, @ performed in the

Raw score (seconds) =
%ile based on Heaton's demographically corrected norms =

Selective Attention: Selective attention refers to the ability to focus attention on one or more relevant aspects of a stimulus or situation while ignoring irrelevant aspects of the stimulus or situation. One way of examining this function is through the use of a Stroop procedure in which subjects are asked to selectively attend to the color of ink that letters are printed in, while ignoring the words they spell. Since reading is such a dominant response to letters grouped in this fashion, mental effort is required to suppress the tendency to read the words. This results in errors and slowing of processing, especially in individuals with reduced selective attention ability. On the Stroop, @ performed in the

Raw number of items correctly answered within 45 seconds =
%ile based on age- and education-corrected norms =

Conclusions Regarding Mental Control: Mental control includes the ability to utilize working memory to place information in temporary storage and retrieve it as needed in performing a task, the ability to flexibly shift attention, and the ability to selectively focus attention in the face of distraction from competing stimuli. Analysis of test performance in this area reveals

LEARNING AND MEMORY FUNCTIONS

Complaints

Self-Report:

Informant Report:

Observational Data: @'s ability to access memory for recent events appeared to be

Test Findings

Orientation: When tested for awareness of basic orientation information, such as time, date, and place, @ performed in the
Cognistat Orientation subtest raw score =

Remote Memory/Fund of Information: Ability to recall the type of information generally learned earlier in life, often from school or family, was assessed with the Wechsler Information subtest. @ scored in the

Raw score =
Scaled score =
%ile for individuals in this age group =

Verbal List Learning: On a test of the ability to learn a list of words presented across several learning trials, @ performed in the

Test: RAVLT
Raw score =
%ile for individuals in this age group =

When asked to recall the list of words after a brief distraction (i.e., exposure to another word list), @ scored in the

Raw number of words recalled =
%ile for individuals in this age group =

When asked to recall the list of words following an approximately 30-minute delay,

@ tested in the
Raw number of words recalled =
%ile for individuals in this age group =

On a recognition task requiring the identification of the words from the original list,

@ scored in the
Words correctly recognized =
%ile for individuals in this age group =
Number of false positives =

Verbal Story Memory: When tested for immediate recall of meaningful verbal information read out loud by the examiner, @ performed in the

Test: Wechsler Memory Scale-IV Logical Memory
Raw score =
%ile for individuals in this age group =

When asked to recall the same narrative information after an approximately half-hour delay, @ performed in the

Raw score =
%ile for individuals in this age group =

Visual Memory: When asked to recall visual-spatial information (in the form of a complex geometric design) after a short delay, @ tested in the
Test: Rey Osterreith Complex Figure Test

Raw score =
%ile for individuals in this age group =

When asked to recall this design after an approximately half-hour delay, @ tested in the

Raw score =
%ile for individuals in this age group =

When asked after a short delay to recall visual-spatial information (in the form of pictures of human and animal interaction), @ tested in the
Test: WMS-III Family Pictures

Raw score =
%ile for individuals in this age group =

When asked to recall these pictures after an approximately half-hour delay, @ tested in the

Raw score =
%ile for individuals in this age group =

Conclusions Regarding Learning and Memory Functions:

COMMUNICATION FUNCTIONS

Complaints

Self-Report:

Informant Report:

Observational Data

Comprehension of Interview Questions and Test Instructions: @'s ability to understand general questions and test instructions appeared

Speech Articulation: Clarity of speech was

Speech Rate and Rhythm: The rate and rhythm with which @ spoke was judged to be

Speech Content: The content of @'s speech was

Nonverbal Aspects of Communication: Nonverbal aspects of communication (e.g., eye contact) appeared to be

Test Findings

Comprehension: When assessed for the ability to understand and respond appropriately to orally presented information, @ performed in the

Cognistat Comprehension raw score =
Complex Ideational Material Test raw score =
Complex Ideational Material Test %ile based on Heaton's demographically corrected norms =

Naming or Word-Finding Ability: On a word-finding task requiring the naming of objects depicted in drawings, @ scored in the

Test: Boston Naming Test
Raw score out of 60 items =
%ile based on Heaton's demographically corrected norms =

Repetition: Ability to repeat phrases immediately after hearing them is sometimes compromised in certain aphasic disorders and can also be compromised by attentional problems. On a repetition task, @ performed in the

Cognistat Repetition subtest raw score =

Reading: On a test of the ability to correctly read individual words of increasing difficulty, @ performed in the

Test: WRAT4
Raw score =

Standard score (based on a mean of 100 and s.d. of 15) =
Grade equivalent =
%ile for individuals in this age group =

Conclusions Regarding Communication Functions:

MOTOR FUNCTIONS

Complaints

Self-Report:

Informant Report:

Observational Data

Handedness:
Ambulation: @ walked

Test Findings

Grip Strength: Grip strength for each hand was measured as the average of two trials with a hand dynamometer.

Dominant hand grip strength tested in the

Average grip strength in kilograms =
%ile based on Heaton's demographically corrected norms =

Nondominant hand grip strength tested in the

Average grip strength in kilograms =
%ile based on Heaton's demographically corrected norms =

Motor Speed: Tapping speed for each hand was measured with the Finger Tapping Test.
Dominant hand speed tested in the

Average number of taps in 10 seconds =
%ile based on Heaton's demographically corrected norms =

Nondominant hand speed tested in the

Average number of taps in 10 seconds =
%ile based on Heaton's demographically corrected norms =

Manual Dexterity: Fine-motor dexterity for each hand was measured by time taken to complete the Grooved Pegboard Test.

Dominant hand dexterity tested in the

# of seconds to complete placement of pegs =
%ile based on Heaton's demographically corrected norms =

Nondominant hand dexterity tested in the

# of seconds to complete placement of pegs =
%ile based on Heaton's demographically corrected norms =

Conclusions Regarding Motor Functions: Compared to individuals of the same gender and similar age and education levels, @ demonstrated

VISUAL-SPATIAL FUNCTIONS

Complaints

Self-Report:

Informant Report:

Observational Data: Performance on visual scanning tasks, double-simultaneous visual stimulation tasks, constructional tasks, and reading tasks was observed for signs of visual neglect, which were
Right-left orientation, observed during visual fields testing, appeared

Screening Results/Test Findings

Near Vision Acuity: Visual acuity with both eyes open was assessed with a pocket vision screener to make certain that @ could adequately perceive test stimuli. Near vision tested as

Acuity = 20/
Corrective lenses:

Visual Fields: Visual fields, screened by confrontation testing, were found to be
Color Vision: Screening for color perception was conducted to ensure that a deficit in this area did not affect test performance. Color vision was found to be
Perception of Visual Detail: Visual alertness, awareness of environmental details, and ability to differentiate essential from nonessential details were assessed with the Wechsler Picture Completion subtest. @ tested in the

Raw score =
Scaled score =

%ile for individuals in this age group =

Visual Scanning Efficiency: Part A of the Trail Making Test requires rapid location of targets on a page, and time taken to complete this task can be used to draw inferences about visual scanning efficiency. @ performed in the

Seconds to complete this task =
%ile based on Heaton's demographically corrected norms =

Sustained Visual Attention: Ability to sustain visual attention and alertness during a tedious clerical task can be inferred from the number of errors made on the Digit Vigilance Test. @ performed in the

Error raw score =
%ile based on Heaton's demographically corrected norms =

Block Design Construction: Spatial analysis and constructional ability were assessed with the Wechsler Block Design task, which requires reproduction of designs of increasing complexity. @ performed in the

Raw score =
Scaled score =
%ile for individuals in this age group =

Drawing Copy: Visual-spatial ability was assessed by having @ attempt to make an accurate copy of a complex design. @ performed in the

Test: Rey Osterreith Complex Figure Test
Copy raw score out of 36 possible points =
%ile for individuals in this age group =

Conclusions Regarding Visual-Spatial Functions: Neuropsychological assessment of visual-spatial functions revealed

OTHER SENSORY-PERCEPTUAL FUNCTIONS

Complaints

Self-Report:
Informant Report:

Observational Data: Ability to hear questions and instructions presented at normal conversational volume appeared to be

Auditory Screening Results/Test Findings

Repetition: Ability to repeat phrases immediately after hearing them provides an indication of whether the subject is able to hear adequately to participate in testing. On a repetition task, @ performed in the
Cognistat Repetition subtest raw score =

Auditory Perception During Single Stimulation: @'s perception of sound made by the examiner lightly rubbing fingers together next to one ear at a time was found to be

Auditory Perception During Double-Simultaneous Stimulation: Unilateral auditory inattention or neglect is sometimes detected by this procedure. @'s ability to detect sound presented simultaneously to each ear was found to be

Auditory Attention Span: Span of auditory attention, measured by number of digits successfully repeated in the forward direction on a digit span task, tested in the

Maximum digits recalled in the forward direction =
Raw score for digits forward =
%ile for individuals in this age group =

Tactile Screening Results

Perception of Single Stimulation: @'s perception of touch presented lightly to one side of the body at a time was found to be

Perception of Double-Simultaneous Stimulation: Unilateral tactile inattention or neglect is sometimes detected by this procedure. @'s ability to detect light touch presented simultaneously to each side of the body was found to be

Discrimination of Shapes: The ability to differentiate simple geometric shapes by touch with each hand was found to be

Finger Recognition: The ability to identify by touch alone the particular finger to which tactile stimulation was applied was found to be

Olfactory Screening Results: Olfactory acuity was assessed with the Quick Smell Identification Test, and @ performed in the

Raw number of smells correctly identified on the 3 screening items =

Conclusions Regarding Other Sensory-Perceptual Functions: On neuropsychological screening, sense of smell was found to be

MENTAL STATUS AND PSYCHOLOGICAL ADJUSTMENT

Presentation and Appearance

Method of Arrival: @
Manner of Presentation/Style of Relating: Compared to other examinees seen in similar contexts, @ was
Appearance: The neatness of dress and grooming appeared

Affect and Mood

Range of Affect: The range of affect displayed by @ appeared

Appropriateness of Affect: The appropriateness of @'s affect to the content of our discussion was judged to be

Level of Depression: Self-reported depression level tested in the

SCL-90-R Depression T-score =
PAI Depression T-score =
HADS Depression raw score =

@'s endorsement or nonendorsement of symptoms that can indicate depression is presented below using this notation system:

	++ = Very True		+= Partly True		Empty = False	

Sadness		Social detachment		Diminished hope		Fatigue/lethargy	
Loss of interest		Failure feelings		Thoughts of death		Excessive sleep	
Loss of enjoyment		Guilt		Reduced self-worth		Impaired sleep maintenance	
Loss of humor		Reduced libido		Diminished will to live		Perceived cognitive problems	
Irritability		Reduced motivation		Restlessness		Appetite changes	
Tearfulness							

Informant report

Clinical interview and behavioral observations

Based on all the data available, I would characterize @ as

Suicidal Ideation:

Irritability:

Level of Anxiety: Self-reported anxiety level tested in the

SCL-90-R Anxiety T-score =
SCL-90-R Phobia T-score =
PAI Anxiety T-score =
PAI Anxiety Related Disorders T-score =
HADS Anxiety raw score =

@'s endorsement or nonendorsement of symptoms that can indicate anxiety is presented below using this notation system:

++ = Very True   **+= Partly True**   **Empty = False**

Worry	Fear of "going crazy"		Social avoidance		Initial insomnia	
Loss of confidence	Phobic fear		Self-consciousness		Muscle tension	
Difficulty relaxing	Phobic avoidance		Repetitive behavior		Perspiration	
Insecurity	Distressing memories/ nightmares		Repetitive thoughts		Breathing/ heart rate change	
Dread	Heightened startle response		Fear of death/loss of control		Appetite/ digestion change	
Panic						

Informant report

Clinical interview and behavioral observations

Muscle tension, assessed with surface EMG, revealed

Device:
Placement:
Microvolts =

Based on all the data available, I would characterize @ as

Behavioral Control, Self-Monitoring, Planning, and Judgment

Initiation: @'s ability to initiate appeared to be

Perseveration: Signs of perseveration were

Impulsivity: Impulsivity was

Self-Monitoring: Self-monitoring to catch and correct errors appeared

Planning: Planning displayed on block-design and drawing tasks was judged to be

Thought Process and Content: @ was also assessed for evidence of delusions, hallucinations, and bizarre or disorganized thinking. Based on this assessment, there is

SCL-90-R Psychoticism T-score =
SCL-90-R Paranoia T-score =
PAI Schizophrenia T-score =
PAI Paranoia T-score =

Self-Awareness: The concordance between @'s self-reported awareness of strengths and weaknesses and actual test results appeared to be

Social and Safety Judgment: Ability to provide appropriate verbal responses to hypothetical commonsense social and safety judgment questions tested in the

Cognistat Judgment subtest raw score =

Personality Assessment Inventory Clinical Interpretive Report

Disclaimer: The Personality Assessment Inventory (PAI) Clinical Interpretive Report presented below is computer generated based on @'s responses to a 344-item measure of personality and psychopathology. This report relies on actuarial data obtained without the benefit of a clinical interview; therefore, the interpretive information presented below should be viewed as only one source of hypotheses about @. These hypotheses are integrated with other data (e.g., from interview and history) in the summary that follows this section. The computer-generated interpretation is presented in smaller font to assist the reader in distinguishing it from the rest of this evaluation.

Validity of Test Results:

Clinical Features:

Self-Concept:

Interpersonal and Social Environment:

Treatment Considerations:

DSM-IV Diagnostic Possibilities:

Conclusions Regarding Mental Status and Psychological Adjustment:

SUMMARY, CONCLUSIONS, AND RECOMMENDATIONS

SUMMARY OF TEST FINDINGS

Overall Assessment of Test Validity:

Intellectual and Problem-Solving Ability:

Processing Speed:

Mental Control:

Learning and Memory Functions:

Communication Functions:

Motor Functions:

Visual-Spatial Functions:

Other Sensory-Perceptual Functions:

Mental Status and Psychological Adjustment:

CONCLUSIONS

What are @'s current areas of neuropsychological and psychological strength and weakness?

Is there evidence of cognitive deficits?

Is there evidence of psychosocial adjustment problems?

What factors, if any, are relevant to causation or apportionment?

Are there other factors, such as pre-existing cognitive problems, poor effort, symptom exaggeration, emotional distress, or chronic pain, that can partially or fully account for any observed cognitive deficits?

What are the vocational or other functional implications of these findings?

Would modifications or adaptations ameliorate these limitations?

What further degree of recovery is expected?

Are there special concerns for @'s future safety or well being?

To what extent is the pattern of current test scores likely due to normal variation, impairment, or other factors?

How do these findings compare to those of previous evaluations?

How can @'s condition best be characterized diagnostically?

Axis I:

Axis II:

Axis III:

Axis IV:

Axis V:

RECOMMENDATIONS

Need for Cognitive Rehabilitation:

Need for Psychological or Psychiatric Treatment:

Need for Future Neuropsychological Testing:

Other Recommendations:

Thank you for this referral. If you have any questions, or if I can be of further assistance. please contact me at ***.

***

Part III
Language

Certain sections of the neuropsychological report are typically more challenging to write than others. In some sections, careful wording is particularly important, as when addressing factors that affect test validity or when describing what tests measure and what results mean. In other sections, clinicians may struggle to generate content, as when formulating treatment recommendations.

The tables below contain sample language that can be used to guide the wording of these sections of your reports. Please keep in mind the need to customize these statements to fit the circumstances of each case. Purchasers of this book may request an editable version of this wording from the author by contacting NeuRules@gmail.com.

Chapter 15
Validity

Section	Topic	Text
Validity		
	Culture/Language	
		@'s linguistic and cultural background did not appear to constitute a barrier to accurate assessment.
		Effort was made to account for the influence of linguistic/cultural factors through careful test selection and interpretation. Even with these precautions, however, evaluation results should be viewed as less definitive and considered only a best available approximation of @'s neuropsychological status. Evaluation by a neuropsychologist with expertise in @'s linguistic/cultural background would be helpful if such a resource is available.
		Care was taken in test selection and in test administration (using an interpreter) to minimize the influence of linguistic and cultural confounds. However, such confounds cannot be totally eliminated, and cultural and linguistic factors were taken into account when interpreting test results.
		It should be clearly acknowledged that @'s limited English proficiency and cultural background limit the validity of this evaluation. However, it should also be noted that one of the two measures on which @ showed evidence of symptom magnification is written in @'s primary language, while the other consists of drawings rather than words.
		Because of reading limitations, the accuracy of @'s responses to self-report measures was verified through interview.
	Emotion	
		@ did not display emotional distress at a level judged to impede test performance.
		@'s ability to focus attention and sustain effort did not appear to be significantly impeded by depression, anxiety, or other emotional factors.

(continued)

R.L. Wanlass, *The Neuropsychology Toolkit: Guidelines, Formats, and Language*,
DOI 10.1007/ 978-1-4614-1882-5_15, © Springer Science+Business Media, LLC 2012

Section	Topic	Text
		Level of psychological distress was assessed in order to gauge whether any such distress was intense enough to be likely to significantly impede @'s ability to focus on test requirements. Based on this assessment, ***.
	General	
		Testing revealed no evidence of malingering of cognitive deficits.
		Test performance may have been compromised to a degree by factors related to ***. However, since these are regular features of @'s life at this point, test results are considered reflective of @'s current level of functioning.
		Prior to the initiation of testing, @ was advised of the importance of giving full effort, and @ agreed to do so. On neuropsychological measures sensitive to effort and motivation, @'s performance suggests that cooperation was ***.
		Potential confounds were taken into account in the selection of test procedures and in the interpretation of test results.
		These factors were taken into account in test selection and interpretation.
		I did not identify issues such as ongoing litigation or application for medical disability that raised suspicion about @'s having motivation to perform poorly; however, @'s scores are poor enough on some validity measures that I would recommend repeat testing if such issues ever do arise.
		Effort exerted on testing appeared to be ***.
		The ability of testing to accurately reflect @'s current status is judged to be ***.
		Consistency of performance across similar tasks was judged to be ***.
		The MMPI-2 is a self-report personality/psychopathology inventory that includes three primary validity scales to help identify exaggeration or minimization of psychopathology. @'s MMPI-2 validity scale profile suggests ***.
		Because @'s performance on the TOMM Trial II was adequate, administration of the TOMM Retention Trial was not necessary.
		The TOMM Trial II and Retention Trial were not necessary to administer due to adequate performance on the TOMM Trial I and on other validity measures.
	Poor Effort	
		I cannot report within a reasonable degree of professional certainty that @ exerted sufficient effort on neuropsychological tests.

(continued)

Section	Topic	Text
		The ability of this testing to accurately reflect @'s current status is judged to be poor due to inconsistent effort, as evidenced by below-passing scores on the majority of test validity measures. The results that follow should be viewed as indicative only of how @ presented on testing. While areas in which @ performed in the normal range can be viewed as valid indicators of at least normal abilities in those areas, test performances that fall below the normal range may underrepresent @'s actual ability level due to insufficient effort on those tests.
		Therefore, results of testing do not likely reflect @'s maximal level of ability.
		Given questions regarding effort and motivation, test results should be viewed as reflecting the manner in which @ presented during testing, but not necessarily indicative of @'s maximal level of functioning.
		Testing of effort and cooperation reveals strong evidence of symptom magnification. The results that follow should be considered to indicate how @ self-presents to others, but are not judged to be reflective of @'s actual level of ability. @'s poor performance on validity measures cannot, in my clinical judgment, be fully explained by other factors such as cultural background, pain, or medication side effects.
		It should be cautioned that the presence of symptom magnification does not rule out the possibility of some genuine underlying pathology. Thus, these test results should not be used as a basis for denying @ authorization for other evaluation procedures that are judged by Dr. *** to be medically indicated.
		The ability of current testing to accurately reflect @'s actual cognitive status is judged to be poor due to failure on *** out of *** effort measures and barely passing scores on the other ***. The possibility of symptom magnification should be strongly considered.
		These test results reflect how @ presented during testing but may not indicate @'s actual level of ability.
		It is possible that there could be some genuine cognitive deficits, but substantial evidence of problems with cooperation/effort places current test results in such doubt that they cannot be interpreted as corroborating @'s cognitive complaints.
		Because @ did not pass *** out of *** validity measures, current test results are unable to substantiate the presence of genuine cognitive deficits.

(continued)

Section	Topic	Text
		Because of questionable performance on validity measures suggesting possible symptom magnification or incomplete effort on testing, these test results cannot be relied upon as being reflective of @'s actual current cognitive and emotional status. Results are provided below to indicate how @ presented on testing, but they should not be construed as necessarily representative of @'s maximal level of performance.
		The large number of items endorsed on the SCL-90-R raises the possibility of a "cry-for-help" profile in which symptoms may have been magnified. However, it is quite common in adversarial situations, such as workers' compensation cases, for patients to over-emphasize their problems out of concern that the distress they genuinely feel will not be recognized or acknowledged. This is especially true when tests and questionnaires are completed prior to meeting with and developing some trust in the examiner, as occurred in this case. Once patients have gained trust in the examiner's objectivity, symptoms are then typically presented without such over-emphasis, unless there is outright malingering, which did not appear to be present in this case. I judge @'s explanations and descriptions of symptoms to be generally credible. I also note that even though @ endorsed a large number (***) of SCL-90-R items, the level of distress assigned to each symptom was not out of the ordinary (PSDI T-score = ***). @ also appeared quite credible during the interview, with nonverbal display of affect consistent with verbal report. The possibility of some over-emphasis of symptoms on measures completed before the clinical interview was taken into account in interpreting scores on those measures.
		The precise degree of psychological distress experienced by @ is difficult to ascertain due to the apparent presence of a "cry for help" profile characterized by possible symptom magnification.
		*** , but questions regarding test validity make it unclear whether there is any actual deficit in this area.
		@ did not appear to be upset by poor performance.
		On memory trials, @ showed inconsistent recognition of the same item.
	Pain/Fatigue	
		With 10 representing the worst imaginable pain and 0 representing no pain, @ reported a pain level of ***.
		On a 0-10 point scale, with 10 representing the worst imaginable pain, @ reported a pain level of *** at the start of testing, with an increase in reported pain level to *** by the end of testing.
		@ did not show outward indications of being in significant pain, however.

(continued)

Section	Topic	Text
		@'s high reported pain level may have contributed to reduced scores, but since @ reported being in a similar level of pain most of the time, test results are likely to reflect @'s typical functioning.
		Regarding fatigue or other physical condition confounds, ***.
		The influence of pain, fatigue, or other physical conditions on ability to concentrate during testing was judged to be ***.
	Medication	
		@ reported having taken *** about *** hours prior to testing. At the time of testing, @ did not appear sedated by medications.
		@ did not appear sedated and did not show evidence of diminished cognitive status due to pain medication.
		@'s medications may have contributed to reduced scores, but since @ takes these medications on an ongoing basis, test results are likely to reflect @'s typical functioning.
		The possibility that medications or substances present in @'s system might affect test performance was considered. Problems of this type were ***.
		No medication confounds were identified.
	Sensorimotor Functions	
		Careful attention was paid to make sure that @ could adequately see and hear stimuli and exercise adequate motor control to respond.
		@ complained of episodic double vision, so I suggested closing or covering of one eye if needed. @ did this on several occasions during testing, but showed no corresponding improvement in accuracy or speed.
		@ complained of episodic double vision, so I suggested closing or covering of one eye if needed. @ did this on several occasions during testing and reported that it helped.
		@'s sensory limitation (***) was taken into account in test selection and interpretation.
		@'s motor limitation (***) was taken into account in test selection and interpretation.
	Practice Effect	
		Practice effect does not appear to be a confound, as I identified no evidence that @ has had prior exposure to these test materials.
		Practice effect does not appear to be a significant confound, as it has been so long (*** years) since @ was exposed to these test materials.
		Practice effect does not appear to be a significant confound, as it has been so long (*** years) since @ was exposed to these test materials and since @'s memory was so impaired at that time.

(continued)

Section	Topic	Text
		@ was previously exposed to neuropsychological test materials (***), which raises the possibility of practice effect artificially raising test performance.
		I attempted to minimize the influence of practice effect from prior test exposure by selecting alternate tests or test versions where possible.
		@ was previously exposed to neuropsychological test materials (***), which raises the possibility of practice effect artificially raising test scores. I attempted to minimize the influence of practice effect from prior test exposure by selecting alternate tests or test versions where possible. Where this was not possible, effort was made to account for the role of practice effect in test interpretation.

Chapter 16
Test Results

Section	Topic	Text
Test Results		
	Intelligence & Problem Solving	
		Records of premorbid cognitive testing were not available.
		@'s level of academic and vocational attainment suggests premorbid functioning in the *** range.
		Performance at word recognition/pronunciation tasks is generally more resistant to decline in the presence of brain impairment than most other cognitive functions and is sometimes used as an indication of premorbid intellectual status. (Such predictions can, however, overestimate the IQ of persons of very low intelligence and underestimate the IQ of persons of very high intelligence. Also, the presence of a pre-existing reading disability obviously reduces the validity of this prediction method.) Using this method, premorbid Full Scale IQ is estimated to have been approximately ***.
		When demographic factors, such as level of education, are combined into the prediction equation along with the reading score, @'s premorbid Full Scale IQ is estimated to have been approximately ***.
		Certain test scores (e.g., Picture Completion, Information) are less likely to show decline in the presence of most types of neurological insult and are therefore viewed as providing information about premorbid status. Results from such "hold" tests suggest that premorbid ability was ***.
		@'s premorbid intellectual ability is estimated to have been ***.

(continued)

R.L. Wanlass, *The Neuropsychology Toolkit: Guidelines, Formats, and Language*,
DOI 10.1007/ 978-1-4614-1882-5_16, © Springer Science+Business Media, LLC 2012

Section	Topic	Text
		Intelligence Quotient: The IQ provides a useful summary score for various abilities that have been defined as constituting "intelligence", or the ability to reason, solve problems, think abstractly, plan, comprehend complex ideas, learn quickly, and learn from experience.
		IQ tests do not assess all of the mental abilities necessary for successful functioning, which is why neuropsychological test batteries include many additional measures.
		It is possible for a person with well-documented brain injury to obtain a normal-range IQ score if pre-injury intellectual ability was above normal or if the injury affected functions not well measured by the IQ test.
		On current testing, @ obtained a Full Scale IQ score of ***.
		Two major components of the Wechsler IQ test are a Verbal Comprehension Index (VCI), measuring verbal comprehension and reasoning ability, and the Perceptual Reasoning Index (PRI), measuring visual-perceptual organization and reasoning ability. Comparison of VCI to PRI reveals ***.
		The General Ability Index (GAI) consists of the Similarities, Vocabulary and Information subtests from the Verbal Comprehension Index and the Block Design, Matrix Reasoning and Visual Puzzles subtests from the Perceptual Reasoning Index. The GAI, therefore, excludes measures of working memory and processing speed and consequently can be clinically useful as a measure of cognitive abilities that are less vulnerable to impairment.
		Verbal Abstraction: On a verbal abstract reasoning task involving the identification of similarities between words, @ scored in the ***.
		Arithmetic Reasoning: Ability to mentally (i.e., with no paper or calculator) solve practical arithmetic problems tested in the ***.
		Nonverbal Reasoning: Ability to solve nonverbal reasoning problems tested in the ***.
		Adaptive Reasoning and Problem Solving: The Category Test has proven to be highly sensitive, often more so than IQ tests, to the reasoning and problem solving deficits that occur after brain injury. This test requires the ability to generate potential solutions to problems, test these in a systematic fashion keeping track of which strategies work and which do not, and adapt flexibly as aspects of the problem change. @ obtained a Category Test score that falls in the ***.

(continued)

Section	Topic	Text
		Performance on the Category Test is considered to be the best representation of an individual's ability to solve the myriad of practical problems of everyday living (Reitan & Wolfson, 1993).
	Processing Speed	
		Observational Data: Mental speed exhibited during several hours of interaction appeared ***.
		Processing Speed on Visual-Motor Tasks: Processing speed can be inferred by rate of completion on a digit-symbol substitution (or "coding") task in which the subject refers to a legend or key to translate numbers into their corresponding symbols. On this task, @ scored in the ***.
		Processing speed can also be inferred by rate of completion on a visual search task in which the subject scans lines as rapidly as possible to detect the presence of matching symbols. On this task, @ scored in the ***.
		Wechsler combines scores on the Coding and Symbol Search tasks into a composite score called the Processing Speed Index (PSI). On this index, @ scored in the ***.
		On a task in which the subject rapidly searches for target symbols among distracting symbols, @ performed in the ***.
		*** but sacrificed accuracy to achieve this score.
		Part A of the Trail Making Test is a connect-the-dot type of task that requires rapid location of targets on a page, and time taken to complete this task can be used to draw inferences about visual scanning speed. @ performed in the ***.
		However, it should be noted that, on the second, more difficult portion of this test (Trails B), @ scored in the normal range, which makes the presence of a significantly reduced visual scanning speed seem unlikely.
		Speed on a simple task requiring the rapid reading of common words (i.e., color names) tested in the ***.
		Speed on a simple task requiring the rapid identification of colors tested in the ***.
		Verbal fluency refers to the ability to generate as many words as possible beginning with a specific letter or falling within a specific category while working under a time limit. This task requires speed in generating new words, preferably utilizing working memory to avoid repetition of words. @ performed in the ***.
		Conclusions Regarding Processing Speed: Analysis of scores on tests of mental speed indicates ***.

(continued)

Section	Topic	Text
	Mental Control	
		Working Memory: Working memory can be defined simply as the memory that holds information we are using at the time.
		One measure of working memory is backward digit recall, which requires the ability to hold information (i.e., a series of numbers) in temporary storage while performing a mental manipulation (i.e., reversal) on it. On the Wechsler digits reverse task, @ scored in the ***.
		The Wechsler Digit Span subtest includes recall of digit sequences in the forward and backward directions, as well as recall of randomly presented digits after mentally rearranging them into numerical order. On this Digit Span task, @ scored in the ***.
		Wechsler's Letter-Number Sequencing (LNS) task requires the examinee to hold a series of randomly ordered letters and numbers in working memory long enough to reorganize them into proper sequence. On this task, @ scored in the ***.
		Wechsler combines scores on the Digit Span and Arithmetic subtests into a composite score called the Working Memory Index (WMI). On this index, @ scored in the ***.
		The Paced Auditory Serial Addition Test (PASAT) requires ability to hold numbers in working memory while rapidly performing simple mental arithmetic as the speed requirement increases across trials. @ obtained a total score that falls in the ***.
		Mental Flexibility/Alternating Attention: Trail Making Test (TMT) Part B is a connect-the-dot type of task that requires the subject to alternate between consecutive numbers and letters as rapidly as possible. On this task, @ performed in the ***.
		Selective Attention: Selective attention refers to the ability to focus attention on one or more relevant aspects of a stimulus or situation while ignoring irrelevant aspects of the stimulus or situation. One way of examining this function is through the use of a Stroop procedure in which subjects are asked to selectively attend to the color of ink that letters are printed in and ignore the words they spell. Since reading is such a dominant response to letters grouped in this fashion, mental effort is required to suppress the tendency to read the words. This results in slowing of processing and errors, especially in individuals with reduced selective attention ability. On the Stroop, @ performed in the ***.

(continued)

Section	Topic	Text
		Conclusions Regarding Mental Control: Mental control includes the ability to utilize working memory to place information in temporary storage and retrieve it as needed in performing a task, the ability to flexibly shift attention, and the ability to selectively focus attention in the face of distraction from competing stimuli. Analysis of test performance in this area reveals ***.
	Learning & Memory	
		Observational Data: @'s ability to access memory for recent events appeared to be ***.
		@ had no apparent difficulty with recall of recent history or of test instructions.
		@ appeared to be a reliable informant regarding recent events.
		Orientation: When tested for awareness of basic orientation information, such as time, date, and place, @ performed in the ***.
		Remote Memory/Fund of Information: Ability to recall the type of information generally learned earlier in life, often from school or family, was assessed with the Wechsler Information subtest. @ scored in the ***.
		Verbal List Learning: On a test of the ability to learn a list of words presented across several learning trials, @ performed in the ***.
		When asked to recall the list of words after a brief distraction (i.e., exposure to another word list), @ scored in the ***.
		When asked to recall the list of words following a 20-30 minute delay, @ tested in the ***.
		On a recognition task requiring the identification of the words from the original list, @ scored in the ***.
		Verbal Story Memory: When tested for immediate recall of meaningful verbal information read out loud by the examiner, @ performed in the ***.
		When asked to recall the same narrative information after an approximately half-hour delay, @ performed in the ***.
		Visual Memory: Recall after a short delay for visual-spatial information (in the form of a complex geometric design) tested in the ***.
		Recall of this design after an approximately half-hour delay tested in the ***.

(continued)

Section	Topic	Text
		Recall after a short delay for visual-spatial information (in the form of pictures of human and animal interaction) tested in the ***.
		Recall of these pictures after an approximately half-hour delay tested in the ***.
	Communication Functions	
		Comprehension of Interview Questions and Test Instructions: @'s ability to understand general questions and test instructions appeared ***.
		Speech Articulation: Clarity of speech was ***.
		Speech Rate and Rhythm: The rate and rhythm with which @ spoke was judged to be ***.
		Speech Content: The content of @'s speech was ***.
		Nonverbal Aspects of Communication: Nonverbal aspects of communication (e.g., eye contact) appeared to be ***.
		Comprehension: When assessed for the ability to listen to, understand, and respond appropriately to orally presented information, @ performed in the ***.
		Naming or Word-Finding Ability: On a word-finding task requiring the naming of objects depicted in drawings, @ scored in the ***.
		Repetition: Ability to repeat phrases immediately after hearing them is sometimes compromised in certain aphasic disorders and can also be compromised by attentional problems. On a repetition task, @ performed in the ***.
		Reading: On a test of the ability to correctly read individual words of increasing difficulty, @ performed in the ***.
	Motor Functions	
		@ walked independently at a normal pace and with no apparent instability.
		Grip Strength: Grip strength for each hand was measured as the average of two trials with a hand dynamometer.
		Dominant (***) hand grip strength tested in the ***.
		Nondominant hand grip strength tested in the ***.
		Motor Speed: Tapping speed for each hand was measured with the Finger Tapping Test.

(continued)

Section	Topic	Text
		Dominant (***) hand speed tested in the ***.
		Nondominant hand speed tested in the ***.
		Manual Dexterity: Fine-motor dexterity for each hand was measured by time taken to complete the Grooved Pegboard Test.
		Dominant (***) hand dexterity tested in the ***.
		Nondominant hand dexterity tested in the ***.
		Conclusions Regarding Motor Functions: Compared to individuals of the same gender and similar age and education levels, @ demonstrated ***.
	Visual-Spatial Functions	
		Observational Data: Performance on visual scanning tasks, double-simultaneous visual stimulation tasks, constructional tasks, and reading tasks was observed for signs of visual neglect, which were ***.
		Right-left orientation, observed during visual fields testing, appeared ***.
		Near Vision Acuity: Visual acuity with both eyes open was assessed with a pocket vision screener to make certain that @ could adequately perceive test stimuli. Near vision tested as ***.
		Visual Fields: Visual fields, screened by confrontation testing, were found to be ***.
		Color Vision: Screening for color perception was conducted to ensure that a deficit in this area did not affect test performance. Color vision was found to be ***.
		Perception of Visual Detail: Visual alertness, awareness of environmental details, and ability to differentiate essential from nonessential details were assessed with the Wechsler Picture Completion subtest. @ tested in the ***.
		Visual Scanning Efficiency: Part A of the Trail Making Test requires rapid location of targets on a page, and time taken to complete this task can be used to draw inferences about visual scanning efficiency. @ performed in the ***.
		Sustained Visual Attention: Ability to sustain visual attention and alertness during a tedious clerical task can be inferred from the number of errors made on the Digit Vigilance Test. @ performed in the ***.

(continued)

Section	Topic	Text
		<u>Block Design Construction</u>: Spatial analysis and constructional ability were assessed with the Wechsler Block Design task, which requires reproduction of designs of increasing complexity. @ performed in the ***.
		Conclusions Regarding Visual-Spatial Functions: Neuropsychological assessment of visual-spatial functions revealed ***.
	Other Sensory-Perceptual Functions	
		Observational Data: Ability to hear questions and instructions presented at normal conversational volume appeared to be ***.
		<u>Repetition</u>: Ability to repeat phrases immediately after hearing them provides an indication of whether the subject is able to hear adequately to participate in testing. On a repetition task, @ performed in the ***.
		<u>Auditory Perception During Single Stimulation</u>: @'s perception of sound made by the examiner lightly rubbing fingers together next to one ear at a time was found to be ***.
		<u>Auditory Perception During Double-Simultaneous Stimulation</u>: Unilateral auditory inattention or neglect is sometimes detected by this procedure. @'s ability to detect sound presented simultaneously to each ear was found to be ***.
		<u>Auditory Attention Span</u>: Span of auditory attention, measured by number of digits successfully repeated in the forward direction on a digit span task, tested in the ***.
		<u>Perception of Single Stimulation</u>: @'s perception of touch presented lightly to one side of the body at a time was found to be ***.
		<u>Perception of Double-Simultaneous Stimulation</u>: Unilateral tactile inattention or neglect is sometimes detected by this procedure. @'s ability to detect light touch presented simultaneously to each side of the body was found to be ***.
		<u>Discrimination of Shapes</u>: The ability to differentiate simple geometric shapes by touch with each hand was found to be ***.
		<u>Finger Recognition</u>: The ability to identify by touch alone the particular finger to which tactile stimulation was applied was found to be ***.

(continued)

Section	Topic	Text
		Olfactory Screening Results: Olfactory acuity was assessed with the Quick Smell Identification Test, and @ performed in the ***.
	Mental Status	
		<u>Manner of Presentation/Style of Relating</u>: Compared to other examinees seen in similar contexts, @ was ***.
		<u>Appearance</u>: The neatness of dress and grooming appeared ***.
		<u>Range of Affect</u>: The range of affect displayed by @ appeared ***.
		<u>Appropriateness of Affect</u>: The appropriateness of @'s affect to the content of our discussion was judged to be ***.
		Affect was appropriate to content but somewhat subdued in range, consistent with mildly depressed mood.
		<u>Level of Depression</u>: Self-reported depression level tested in the ***.
		@ did not demonstrate euphoria, grandiosity, pressured speech, or flight of ideas that would reflect the presence of mania or hypomania.
		@ reported being depressed, but did not outwardly appear depressed.
		*** suggests anxiety and depression at a more mild level than indicated on self-report measures.
		Mood will likely improve once @ is physically able to resume gainful activity and recreational pursuits.
		@'s endorsement or nonendorsement of symptoms that can indicate depression is presented below using this notation system:

++ = Very True   **+ = Partly True**   **Empty = False**

Sadness	Social detachment	Diminished hope	Fatigue/ lethargy
Loss of interest	Failure feelings	Thoughts of death	Excessive sleep
Loss of enjoyment	Guilt	Reduced self-worth	Impaired sleep maintenance
Loss of humor	Reduced libido	Diminished will to live	Perceived cognitive problems
Irritability	Reduced motivation	Restlessness	Appetite changes
Tearfulness			

Section	Topic	Text
		<u>Level of Anxiety</u>: Self-reported anxiety level tested in the ***.
		@'s endorsement or nonendorsement of symptoms that can indicate anxiety is presented below using this notation system: **++ = Very True + = Partly True Empty = False**

Worry	Fear of "going crazy"	Social avoidance	Initial insomnia
Loss of confidence	Phobic fear	Self-consciousness	Muscle tension
Difficulty relaxing	Phobic avoidance	Repetitive behavior	Perspiration
Dread	Distressing memories/ nightmares	Repetitive thoughts	Breathing/ heart rate change
Panic	Heightened startle response	Fear of death/loss of control	Appetite/ digestion change

Section	Topic	Text
		Posttraumatic stress disorder (PTSD) symptoms are considered less common in cases of traumatic brain injury than in cases of other types of trauma because the impact to the brain in traumatic brain injury often interferes with the formation of memory for the events surrounding the injury. However, there are cases in which the injured individual did form a memory of stressful events surrounding the injury and did experience intense fear associated with threatened or actual serious harm. Therefore, it is important in such cases to assess for possible symptoms of PTSD.
		<u>Initiation</u>: @'s ability to initiate appeared to be ***.
		<u>Perseveration</u>: Signs of perseveration were ***.
		<u>Impulsivity</u>: Impulsivity was ***.
		<u>Self-Monitoring</u>: Self-monitoring to catch and correct errors appeared ***.
		<u>Planning</u>: Planning displayed on block-design and drawing tasks was judged to be ***.
		<u>Thought Process and Content</u>: @ was also assessed for evidence of delusions, hallucinations, and bizarre or disorganized thinking. Based on this assessment, ***.
		There is no evidence from clinical interview of confusion, psychosis, medication-induced sedation, or other signs of diminished mental status.

(continued)

Section	Topic	Text
		@ did not make any comments or exhibit any behaviors suggestive of delusional thinking or hallucinatory experience.
		During several hours of testing and interview, @ did not report or exhibit delusions, hallucinations, loose associations, bizarre mental content, or other signs of psychosis.
		@ demonstrated linear and coherent thought, and there is no evidence of psychosis or other gross disturbance in mentation.
		Self-Awareness: The concordance between @'s self-reported awareness of strengths and weaknesses and actual test results appeared to be ***.
		Social and Safety Judgment: Ability to provide appropriate verbal responses to hypothetical commonsense social and safety judgment questions tested in the ***.
		Personality Assessment Inventory Clinical Interpretive Report
		The Personality Assessment Inventory (PAI) Clinical Interpretive Report presented below is computer generated based on @'s responses to a 344-item measure of personality and psychopathology. This report relies on actuarial data obtained without the benefit of a clinical interview; therefore, the interpretive information presented below should be viewed as only one source of hypotheses about @. These hypotheses are integrated with other data (e.g., from interview and history) in the summary that follows this section. The computer-generated interpretation is presented in smaller font to assist the reader in distinguishing it from the rest of this evaluation.

Chapter 17
Conclusions

Section	Topic	Text
Conclusions		
	Impaired	
		Problems of this type are common following closed-head injury, and in the absence of other explanatory factors and absence of a history of problems of this type prior to the injury, the closed-head injury @ sustained on *** is judged to be the most likely cause of these problems.
		Absent evidence to the contrary and based on information available to me at this time, it does appear that @'s complaints are related to the injury as described.
	Impaired but…	
		@'s cognitive test performance is somewhat atypical for persons with mild TBI in that @ did so well on *** tasks, so it is not clear whether the cognitive deficits are pre-existing or due to the injury. Dr. ***, or another medical expert, may be able to correlate these findings with other diagnostic findings to reach a clearer conclusion regarding the etiology of the cognitive problems @ demonstrates.
		@'s subjective complaints significantly exceed expectations based on estimates of injury severity.
	Normal	
		Testing does not provide objective evidence of residual cognitive deficits from the injury.

(continued)

R.L. Wanlass, *The Neuropsychology Toolkit: Guidelines, Formats, and Language,* 129
DOI 10.1007/ 978-1-4614-1882-5_17, © Springer Science+Business Media, LLC 2012

Section	Topic	Text
		It should be noted that healthy, uninjured persons who are given a large battery of tests typically do not score in the normal range on all tests. Some variability in performance is expected. As noted by Heaton, Grant, & Matthews in their Revised Comprehensive Norms for an Expanded Halstead-Reitan Battery (2004), "some poor test results are to be expected in most normal persons, especially when a large battery of tests is administered." They also state that, "it is a serious mistake to assume that one or more test scores beyond the accepted cutoff scores always indicate the presence of an acquired cerebral disorder." By my counting, @ had *** scores in the range that Heaton et al. would consider impaired out of *** cognitive test scores. This is not out of the expected range for neurologically normal subjects, as indicated in the Heaton et al. book.
	Normal but...	
		While it is possible that @ has experienced a decline in *** functioning from an above-normal pre-injury ability level, there is no way to establish that scientifically in the absence of pre-injury neuropsychological test data showing that @ was, in fact, well above normal in those areas.
		@ has recovered very well from any cognitive sequelae that may have occurred following the injury. @ continues to demonstrate a high level of cognitive ability across most areas assessed, and there is no test-based evidence of cognitive impairment. It is, of course, possible that some subtle cognitive changes could have occurred at a level below the threshold detectable by cognitive testing in such an intellectually superior individual, but the reported lack of more than momentary alteration in consciousness at the time of the accident makes this less likely.
		Even in the absence of a cognitive disorder, momentary disruption in concentration due to pain, fatigue, distraction, or stress associated with the accident can result in occasional lapses in mental efficiency.
		There may, however, be episodes of reduced concentration in @'s daily life due to one or more of these factors: pain, fatigue, preoccupation with problems, medication side effects, emotional distress. These episodes of reduced concentration may result in instances of cognitive ineffi-ciency such as poor memory for specific events to which @ was not paying close attention due to the factors noted above.
		It is possible, of course, that some subtle cognition changes could have occurred at a level below the threshold detectable by cognitive testing in such an intellectually superior individual, but the reported lack of significant alteration in consciousness at the time of the accident makes this less likely.

(continued)

Section	Topic	Text
		It is clear from the medical records that @ did suffer a *** injury, but neuropsychological test data indicate a remarkable degree of recovery. @ currently shows many very considerable cognitive strengths, including above normal performance in some areas typically found to be sensitive to the effects of brain injury (e.g., ***). At this point in @'s recovery, there is no clear indication of residual cognitive impairment. It is, of course, possible that these are some areas in which @ has declined from a premorbidly superior range to the normal range, but this cannot be documented in the absence of pre-injury neuropsychological testing.
		The possibility should be acknowledged that @'s perception of diminished higher cognitive ability could be accurate and that neuropsychological testing is just not sensitive enough to demonstrate the subtle residual deficits. This can be the case when someone who premorbidly was far above normal declines to the normal range after a neurological event. In the absence of premorbid neuropsychological testing, such changes can go undetected.
		It is also acknowledged that some uninjured persons demonstrate as much variability in performance on cognitive testing as @ did, so it is certainly possible that @'s pattern of scores just represents normal variation. This is a difficult call to make in @'s case, but I think it is reasonable to give the benefit of the doubt to the injured worker and allow @ some brief cognitive rehabilitation therapy.
		@ appeared to be putting forth good effort and cooperation during testing, and results appear to be a valid reflection of @'s cognitive ability insofar as it can be tested in a laboratory setting. The reader is, however, cautioned that neuropsychological testing is, by nature, very structured and controlled to reduce variance and enhance measurement precision. An unintended but unfortunate consequence of this structure, however, is that we do not see in the testing lab how a person's performance might change if, for example, the person became stressed, experienced a change in blood sugar or, through a lapse in concentration, took too much or too little medication. Thus, reviewers of this report are urged to recognize the limitations of this type of formalized, structured testing and also take into account reports of healthcare providers and others about how well @ is able to function and how much supervision or assistance @ requires under real-life conditions.
	Vocational implications	
		No cognitive or emotional barriers to work re-entry were identified.
		In fact, work would probably be beneficial for @'s mood and self-esteem as long as it is not overly stressful, and @ is allowed the flexibility to rest when in pain or fatigued.

(continued)

Section	Topic	Text
		It should be noted, however, that normal-range performance for persons aged *** in areas of functioning such as memory is not the same as normal-range performance for younger adults. For example, if @'s delayed word list recall were judged using norms from *** year olds with @'s same level of education, @'s performance would only fall at the ***%ile.
		Therefore, for @ to compete in the workforce, I recommend continued use of the memory strategies developed in cognitive rehabilitation with ***.
		On the other hand, years of experience in a career, wisdom about how to prioritize and work efficiently, and well-developed interpersonal networks on the job can help to mitigate the effects of decline in areas such as memory and processing speed, and it is expected that this will be the case for @.

Chapter 18
Recommendations

Section	Topic	Text
Recommendations		
	Cooperation	
		Provision of increased structure and consistency in @'s environment should decrease anxiety and confusion and lead to improved cooperation.
		Family and healthcare providers should avoid fostering excessive helplessness and dependency by doing too much for @. Instead, they should gradually increase @'s responsibilities while providing necessary structure, guidance, and encouragement. Social reinforcement should be provided contingent upon progress and effort towards independence.
		Cooperation in therapy can be enhanced by starting with more enjoyable (or at least less unpleasant) tasks to build rapport.
		Cooperation in therapy can be enhanced by offering some choice over therapy tasks and the order with which they are performed.
		Cooperation in therapy can be enhanced by allowing brief ventilation about grievances (e.g., perceived poor treatment). Show empathic understanding and validate the normalcy of @'s feelings without inappropriately undermining others at whom @ may be angry.
		Cooperation in therapy can be enhanced by explaining the purpose of treatment in terms of working toward @'s own personal goals (e.g., this will help you drive/walk/get out of the hospital/***).

(continued)

R.L. Wanlass, *The Neuropsychology Toolkit: Guidelines, Formats, and Language*,
DOI 10.1007/ 978-1-4614-1882-5_18, © Springer Science+Business Media, LLC 2012

Section	Topic	Text
		Cooperation in therapy can be enhanced by breaking complex tasks into smaller steps and offering praise for completion of each step. Add additional steps only after mastery of the previous step has been achieved.
		Cooperation in therapy can be enhanced by designing treatment around premorbid interests /activities (i.e., rather than blaming @ for being uncooperative, assume it is the therapist's responsibility for making treatment activities motivating, relevant, fun, etc).
		Cooperation in therapy can be enhanced by appealing to @'s sense of altruism by requesting assistance in working with another patient (as long as this does not present a risk of harm to the other patient, and confidentiality standards are maintained).
		If @ refuses an important activity, do not argue or insist. Instead, change the subject and reintroduce the activity later when rapport is stronger.
		If @ has taken a stand against performing some treatment activity and it would cause loss of face to back down, offer a way out that will allow face saving (e.g., compromise).
		Cooperation in therapy can be enhanced by making sure that @ is not being treated in a condescending fashion (e.g., talked about as if not present or able to understand, or addressed as a child or feeble-minded person).
		Cooperation in therapy can be enhanced by selectively rewarding effort and compliance (i.e., give praise, attention, or other rewards immediately after compliance and withdraw these after noncompliance). Avoid coaxing or other potentially reinforcing attention in response to refusal, since this may increase the likelihood of future refusal.
		Cooperation in therapy can be enhanced by assigning treatment staff members who have the best working relationship with @.
		Cooperation in therapy can be enhanced by establishing behavioral contracts with clearly defined objectives (e.g., walk 200 feet per treatment session) and clearly specified, highly motivating, and promptly delivered rewards. Rewards can be identified by interviewing @ or the family about premorbid activities/interests or by observing @'s behavior (e.g., if @ watches TV or plays video games whenever possible, then these activities may serve as powerful incentives or rewards).

(continued)

Section	Topic	Text
		If rewards cannot be given immediately after an activity, use "token" (e.g., points/play money/certificates) that can be accumulated and exchanged for rewards.
		Cooperation in therapy can be enhanced by designing treatment activities to be successful about 80% of the time so that @ is not overwhelmed by the recognition of deficits.
		Cooperation in therapy can be enhanced by using a 4:1 ratio of praise to criticism (but be careful to praise in a manner that will not be perceived as condescending).
	Aggression	To better manage aggression, reward @ for exercising self-control or otherwise exhibiting behavior incompatible with aggression.
		To better manage aggression, do not actively punish aggression since this usually leads to increased hostility.
		To better manage aggression, withdraw attention or other reinforcers immediately following aggression.
		To better manage aggression, be careful not to inadvertently reward aggressive outbursts by increasing attention in an attempt to calm or reassure @ (if such attention is reinforcing).
		To better manage aggression, determine environmental precipitants to aggression (e.g., excessive noise or other stimulation, unnecessary restraints, lack of structure and consistency) and decrease these triggering factors.
		To better manage aggression, remain calm to avoid escalation of @'s aggression and do not take attacks personally.
		To better manage aggression, provide a high ratio of success experiences. This approach may reduce the likelihood of intense emotional or behavioral reaction precipitated by confrontation with one's deficits.
		To better manage aggression, attempt to redirect @'s attention away from the source of irritation.
		To better manage aggression, do not physically "corner" @ or otherwise make @ feel trapped.
		To minimize irritability related to disorientation and confusion: 1. provide orientation information frequently 2. maintain a constant and structured environment (e.g., do not change rooms unnecessarily) 3. bring in familiar objects from home 4. invite familiar people to participate in treatment 5. design treatment around familiar activities.

(continued)

Section	Topic	Text
		To better manage aggression, have an adequate number of staff available to prevent harm to @ or the staff.
		To better manage aggression, teach @ cognitive and behavioral strategies for controlling anger. These strategies may include learning to recognize actions and thoughts that seem to trigger anger and developing alternative actions (e.g., assertiveness, leaving situations, muscle relaxation, deep breathing) and alternative thoughts (e.g., lowering expectations, considering other interpretations, employing distracting or humorous thoughts).
		@'s medical doctor(s) may wish to consider the advisability of trying one of the medications (e.g., carbamazepine, propranolol, lithium) that have been reported to be effective in treating anger problems following TBI.
	Emotional Lability	If @ demonstrates affective lability that appears to be associated with a grief response, acknowledge @'s sense of loss and validate the appropriateness of these feelings and their expression.
		Some patients experience reduction in tearfulness associated with brain injury-related "emotional incontinence" following initiation of SSRI medication, even in the absence of a diagnosable level of clinical depression.
		In responding to @'s affective lability, briefly acknowledge that after brain injury a person sometimes has less control over emotions for a while and that it is not a sign of weakness, although you understand that it can be embarrassing. Then do not attend or comment further about affective lability.
	Agitation	To reduce agitation, use calm, soft speech and slow movements.
		To reduce agitation, reduce environmental stimuli (e.g., TV, excessive activity in room, multiple visitors).
		To reduce agitation, keep the treatment staff and the environment as consistent as possible.
		To reduce agitation, incorporate orientation information (e.g., date, location) into conversation.
		To reduce agitation, have the family bring in some of @'s personal items to make the environment seem more familiar.
		To reduce agitation, prior to initiating treatment or nursing interventions, address @ by name and describe what you are about to do.
		Educate staff and family about the nature of agitation so that they do not take @'s behavior or comments personally.

(continued)

Section	Topic	Text
		If @ becomes upset about something, redirect @'s attention.
		Caution is recommended in prescribing neuroleptics to Rancho Level IV agitated patients as such medications may impede recovery and may intensify the confusion that is contributing to agitated behavior.
		Explain to family and treatment staff that Rancho Level IV agitation is a sign of continuing progress and is generally time limited.
		Pain coping can be improved by using distraction (e.g., have a talk about something interesting, play music, turn on TV) during uncomfortable therapy activities.
		Pain coping can be improved by providing @ an endpoint (e.g., "We need to do this ten times") to therapy exercises.
	Driving	
		Overall, test results raise a number of concerns about the cognitive abilities underlying safe operation of a motor vehicle.
		An on-the-road driving test by an occupational therapist who specializes in driving evaluations or by a qualified driving instructor is recommended due to safety concerns identified on testing (e.g., ***).
		Resumption of driving is not recommended at this time because of concerns identified in testing, including ***.
	Education	
		A more in-depth educational evaluation is recommended to thoroughly assess @'s academic strengths and weaknesses
		Problems in the ability to comprehend and remember written material can be partially compensated for through the use of the "SQ3R" method. This method includes five steps, the first of which is to survey the written material to gain a general overview of what topics are covered and how they are organized. The second step involves the formulation of specific questions that one hopes to have answered through careful reading of the material. After the initial survey and formulation of questions, the material is read and then recited or rehearsed in one's own words. Written notes of the main points can be made. The material should then be reviewed one last time to remind oneself of the "big picture" as well as how specific bits of information relate to it. Although this approach will require more time and effort, especially initially, it will likely result in significantly better reading comprehension and recall.

(continued)

Section	Topic	Text
		Instruction in basic study skills and time management could improve @'s efficiency in the academic environment.
		@ will learn new information more slowly than before the brain injury and will, therefore, need to study harder. To counteract the inevitable frustration that @ will feel, family and teachers should provide abundant encouragement and praise for effort. @ should be discouraged from comparing current performance to premorbid levels and, instead, encouraged to focus on degree of improvement since the brain injury.
		Individual attention and supplementary instruction will be needed because of @'s problems with attention, memory and organization.
		Because of attentional problems, it will be difficult for @ to both take notes and listen carefully to what the teacher is saying. Therefore, arrangements should be made to obtain notes from the teacher or a classmate or to use an audio recorder so that @ can focus exclusively on what the teacher is saying.
		In resuming academic coursework, @ should begin with a light course load in order to allow gradual readjustment to the academic environment.
		Because of @'s outward appearance of physical health, teachers may underestimate the degree of @'s cognitive impairment. It will be helpful for @'s teachers to be educated about the nature of @'s problems so that they can closely monitor progress and make necessary adjustments to @'s educational program.
		Attentional problems in school can be reduced by seating @ near the front of the room close to the teacher, but away from sources of distraction such as windows or doors.
		Attentional problems in school can be reduced if a screened-off work area can be provided to further minimize distractions when @ is performing particularly challenging assignments.
		The use of brief, clearly explained tasks that have a well-defined endpoint will help @ maintain focus.
		To reduce attentional problems, @ should receive social reinforcement for on-task behavior, with special care being taken not to inadvertently reinforce inappropriate or off-task behavior.
		If social reinforcement is not potent enough to elicit appropriate on-task behavior, consideration should be given to the development of a token-economy program.

(continued)

Section	Topic	Text
		It appears that @ has the potential to manage community college-level coursework. However, this should be attempted on a gradual basis with assistance of the college's disabled students' counseling services to help select appropriate courses.
		@ would benefit from remedial coursework in math/spelling/reading/study skills/ ***.
		The results of this evaluation should be communicated to @'s school for use in educational planning.
		With the written consent of ***, a copy of this evaluation is being provided to @'s school for use in educational planning.
		We would be pleased to work with the school system to facilitate @'s successful integration into the academic environment.
	Family	
		@'s family would benefit from education about the need for establishing clear rules and firm behavioral limits and the importance of attending to and rewarding positive (rather than negative) behaviors.
		@'s family should be encouraged to focus on @'s ongoing progress since injury rather than continually comparing present status to premorbid level of functioning.
		@'s family should be reassured that their own feelings are normal and appropriate given the highly stressful family situation. A family support group (e.g., ***) may be helpful in showing them that they are not alone in their experience.
		The family should be referred to the ***, which provides support groups for head injured survivors and family members.
		It is recommended that @ be referred to *** for family therapy.
		It is recommended that @'s family be provided with detailed information about @'s current status and training in how to interact to maximize @'s recovery and adaptation. The family should be provided with a realistic appraisal of prognosis and be encouraged to take appropriate steps to plan for the changes that @'s residual deficits will cause in the family structure.
		The family should be helped to locate appropriate support and respite care to minimize the risk of burnout as they care for @.

(continued)

Section	Topic	Text
		The adjustment of @'s children to the injury should also be assessed, with referrals made for counseling as appropriate.
		While @'s family is to be commended for their willingness to provide care, they need to be aware that an overly solicitous approach to chronic pain problems may result in an inadvertent reinforcement of pain preoccupation and disability status.
	General	
		Fatigue is likely to magnify @'s neuropsychological deficits; therefore, @ should be urged to obtain adequate rest and sleep, as well as to maintain an adequate nutritional intake.
		No further psychological or neuropsychological intervention appears to be necessary at this time; however, @ was advised to contact us in the future if concerns or problems in adaptation arise.
		I have scheduled a feedback session with @ and will present all of these recommendations at that time.
		Re-evaluation in one year is recommended to assess the extent of recovery and assist in making appropriate plans for future rehabilitation and/or education.
	Language	
		@ will require ongoing feedback from others to improve clarity of speech.
		Because of language comprehension problems, information should be presented in a clear, succinct, but not condescending, fashion.
		Because of deficient auditory-verbal comprehension, gestures and demonstrations should be used to facilitate communication.
		A thorough audiological exam is recommended, as hearing difficulties may be contributing to communication problems.
		Consultation with a speech-language pathologist is recommended to address @'s expressive/receptive communication problems.
		@ should be encouraged to use the technique of paraphrasing to verify proper understanding of what others say. This technique will also facilitate @'s memory for that material.
	Rehab	
		@ would benefit from a structured head injury rehabilitation program such as ***.

(continued)

Section	Topic	Text
		@ would benefit from a structured day treatment program specializing in brain injury rehabilitation, such as the ***. If participation in a brain injury day treatment program is not possible, outpatient services (e.g., neuropsychology, occupational therapy, speech pathology) would be useful for remediating functional and cognitive deficits and facilitating psychosocial adaptation to residual limitations.
		@ should be encouraged to participate in hobbies or other activities that involve manipulation of objects in order to improve manual dexterity.
		@ is likely to benefit from cognitive rehabilitation for problems with ***. It is recommended that @ be referred to *** for these services, which are expected to require *** sessions.
		@ would likely benefit from therapy activities designed to gradually increase awareness of deficits and their implications and facilitate the acquisition of compensatory strategies and the development of realistic plans for the future. This will need to be done within a supportive, reinforcing environment in order to maintain self-esteem and motivation.
		Left-sided visual neglect should be addressed through the use of training materials with bold, brightly colored left margins. @ should be trained in scanning to the left of these materials until locating the bold border.
		One of @'s most significant functional deficits is in the area of memory. @ should be trained in the use of external aids to help compensate for memory deficits. Specifically, @ should be taught to use an appointment book (or "memory log") to record future plans to compensate for prospective memory deficits. @ should also be taught to use this "memory log" as a journal or diary to record notes about what happened each day. The process of writing this information and reviewing it several times will help @ to remember what happened. It would also be helpful for this book to include telephone numbers and addresses, as well as personal information to which @ will need ready access (e.g., health insurance information). Because of the likelihood that @ will lose this portable "memory log," it is also a good idea to keep a backup book in a safe place at home. Each day the information added to the portable book should be re-recorded in the back-up book. The extra review involved in rewriting this information will also help with memory for past and future events.

(continued)

Section	Topic	Text
		@ may also benefit from the use of other memory aids such as a cell phone with calendar, alarm, and voice memo functions. Other options include an alarm wristwatch and an audio recorder, but, whatever the device, @ will need training and practice.
		@ should also be instructed in how to process new information actively rather than passively to increase retention.
		The use of lists posted in the environment may help @ recall the correct sequence for performing necessary activities of daily living.
		For each of these interventions, considerable attention will be needed to insure that these skills are generalized beyond the treatment setting.
		@ should be advised to contact the *** at *** to become involved in a peer support group.
		@ should be advised to contact the Brain Injury Association at (800) 444-6443 or http://www.biausa.org/ for information about the nearest available peer support group.
		@ should be advised to participate in one of the local support groups for stroke survivors. Information about these groups can be obtained by contacting *** at ***.
		Involvement in a health club or organized sports or fitness program may benefit @ by increasing social contacts and improving mood and self-esteem. Medical clearance should be obtained prior to such involvement, however.
		Involvement in low-stress volunteer activities may benefit @ by increasing social contacts and improving mood and self-esteem. Information has been/should be/will be provided to @'s family on how to contact resources that link volunteers to available openings such as volunteermatch.org.
		According to the 1998 NIH Consensus Statement on cognitive rehabilitation: "Cognitive exercises, including computer-assisted strategies, have been used to improve specific neuropsychological processes, predominantly attention, memory, and executive skills. Both randomized controlled studies and case reports have documented the success of the interventions using intermediate outcome measures. Certain studies using global outcome measures also support the use of computer-assisted exercises in cognitive rehabilitation."

(continued)

Section	Topic	Text
		Some improvement can be expected with cognitive rehabilitation therapy. Sessions are usually conducted for one hour two to three times a week, and I would recommend *** sessions.
	Safety	
		@ appears to require distant/close/24-hour/*** supervision in order to ensure safety and well-being.
		Specific areas of concern in this regard are the potential for mismanagement of finances/ the potential for mismanagement of medication or other aspects of health care/ the risk of becoming lost/ the risk of being taken advantage of by others/ the risk of endangering self or others through deliberate/ impulsive acts/ the potential for substance abuse/ and ***.
		@ should be cautioned to avoid hazardous activities and to exercise extra safety precautions, as the effects of repeated brain injuries can be cumulative.
		@ showed no indication during the evaluation of a need for supervision by others. However, since the testing environment is quite structured, family members should observe @ in less structured situations to satisfy themselves that @ is, in fact, capable of functioning safely without supervision.
		Due to impulsivity/poor problem-solving ability/ inattention/ forgetfulness/ lack of deficit awareness and ***, @ may not always exercise sound judgment in real life situations; continued supervision is, therefore, recommended.
		@ should receive extensive instruction and rehearsal in how to respond appropriately to police, fire, or medical emergency.
		@ should be prohibited from operating potentially dangerous equipment or machinery.
		@ should be closely supervised when operating potentially dangerous equipment or machinery.
		Because of @'s judgment limitations, consultation with an objective, trusted relative or other advisor is recommended prior to making important life decisions.
	Work	
		Although not appropriate at this time for vocational re-entry, @ should be re-evaluated in six months/one year/ *** to reassess neuropsychological readiness for work re-entry.

(continued)

Section	Topic	Text
		@ appears to be *** motivated to return to work but is, in my opinion, unable to safely resume previous job duties.
		@ appears to be *** motivated to return to work but is, in my opinion, not yet capable of attaining or maintaining competitive employment.
		It is my expectation that @'s inability to work competitively will last at least one year from the date of the injury/ will be permanent/ will last for ***.
		@ appears to be capable of returning to work.
		Referral for vocational rehabilitation does not appear to be warranted at this time.
		Referral to *** for vocational rehabilitation services appears to be warranted at this time. I have instructed @ in how to initiate this contact by calling *** and encouraged @ to do so.
		@ should be advised to avoid work environments involving exposure to potentially hazardous situations requiring rapid decision-making and response/***.
		It is recommended that @ return to work on a part-time basis and build back up to full-time work only as stamina and frustration tolerance allow.
		@ will probably function best in a work setting that is structured and routine in nature and that allows for frequent feedback and encouragement from an understanding supervisor.
		In planning for work re-entry, care will need to be taken to avoid job sites where @'s limitations will pose a risk to @'s safety or the safety of others.
		It may be psychologically difficult for @ to accept employment at reduced pay or status. Psychological intervention may be needed to assist in ventilating feelings of anger, shame, and sadness over this loss of vocational status. @ should then be helped to compare current status to the level of functioning immediately after the injury. In this way, @ can begin to focus more on the progress than on the losses.
		@ will function best in a work environment with few distractions.
		@ will require frequent breaks during work activity to minimize fatigue and associated reduction in speed and quality of performance.
		For those tasks that cannot be structured in advance by a supervisor, @ should be trained to first plan out the necessary steps to take and then to carefully monitor performance quality. Such training will be most effective if carried out in a job setting that closely approximates @'s eventual job placement.

(continued)

Section	Topic	Text
	Substance Use	
		All treatment staff and family members should provide @ with a consistent message regarding reduced tolerance for alcohol or other drugs and risk that use of such substances may cause serious medical complications (e.g., seizures, dangerous interactions with prescribed medications), inhibit the natural healing process of the brain, intensify emotional and behavioral problems, and increase the risk of further injury to the brain.
		@ should be strongly encouraged to seek available resources (e.g., Alcoholics Anonymous/Narcotics Anonymous/***) to help control the temptation to resume substance abuse.
		Since @'s social life has previously revolved to a large extent around substance use, @ will need assistance in exploring alternative social and recreational opportunities.
		Family members and friends should be encouraged to serve as positive role models by avoiding excessive alcohol consumption and use of illegal drugs.
		@'s family should set limits regarding alcohol and drug use, with clearly identified consequences.
		@'s current pattern of substance use appears to be excessive and maladaptive in terms of its impact upon functioning. @ should be encouraged to avoid substance use and seek treatment for this problem.
	Suicide Risk	
		Because of @'s suicidal ideation, mental health intervention is recommended to reduce emotional distress and to monitor suicide risk and need for hospitalization.
		@ should be considered a potential suicide risk based on the presence of suicidal ideation/suicide plan/ suicide plan and means to carry out this plan/ previous history of a suicide attempt/ previous history of multiple suicide attempts/ significant depression/ hopelessness/ impulsivity/poor problem solving/ limited social support/ ***.
		@ has agreed that prior to attempting suicide or self-harm, @ will contact ***.
		@'s family should be advised to remove lethal items (e.g., weapons, hazardous medications and chemicals) from access and to monitor @'s mood and behavior for signs of increased suicidality.

(continued)

Section	Topic	Text
		@'s family should also be advised that they should contact law enforcement if they believe that @ is imminently suicidal but is unwilling to go for help voluntarily.
	Pain	
		EMG biofeedback can be used to learn to relax chronically tense muscles that may be exacerbating @'s pain. Biofeedback may also increase appreciation for the role played by chronic muscle tension in maintaining pain and thereby strengthen @'s motivation to apply tension reduction strategies on a regular basis.
		Biofeedback frequently has the further benefit of reaffirming patients' sense of control over their physical functioning, which can counteract the sense of helplessness that often accompanies chronic pain.
		@ may benefit from a treatment approach emphasizing the development of behavioral (e.g., muscle relaxation, diaphragmatic breathing) and cognitive (e.g., visualization, self-hypnosis, distraction, reinterpretation) pain management strategies.
		I recommend training in stress management techniques to reduce the stress that may be exacerbating @'s pain.
		@ may benefit from behavioral self-management training to increase compliance with recommended treatment.
		@ may benefit from modification of expectations regarding a pain "cure" and encouragement to adopt more realistic expectations (e.g., to minimize the impact of pain and maximize the effectiveness of coping strategies).
		I provided @ with some initial orientation to physiological self-regulation (e.g., EMG biofeedback, diaphragmatic breathing) for tension reduction, as well as cognitive behavioral techniques for self-management of depressed mood, irritability, and maladaptive cognitions. It would be helpful, however, for @ to receive some additional psychological treatment to increase and improve these skills.
		Short-term psychological pain management therapy can be helpful. Commonly this treatment can be accomplished in fewer than 10 sessions. Treatment that emphasizes self-management of pain will be most effective.

(continued)

Section	Topic	Text
		I recommend 5-6 sessions of individual pain management training incorporating biofeedback, relaxation training, imagery, self-hypnosis, and related cognitive-behavioral intervention to increase @'s ability to self-regulate pain and associated emotional distress.
		The goal of this treatment will be to strengthen @'s pain coping skills through training in a variety of cognitive-behavioral techniques such as muscle relaxation, diaphragmatic breathing, imagery/self-hypnosis, cognitive restructuring, sleep regulation, activity pacing, attentional diversion, mood self-regulation, and adoption of a more internal locus of control.
		If @ does not show adequate involvement in and response to pain self-management intervention, the duration of planned treatment may be shortened.
		@ would likely benefit from training in pain management (e.g., training in distraction techniques, pain signal reinterpretation, mental imagery, muscle relaxation, deep breathing, or self-hypnosis).
		The psychometric testing profile indicates the presence of enough symptoms related to depression to warrant consideration of treatment with antidepressant medication. Medical research has shown that antidepressants can not only be helpful with treating symptoms of depression, but also be useful in the treatment of the pain/sleep disturbance cycles associated with chronic pain.
		Prescription of habituating pain medications should be done with considerable caution since assessment results suggest that @ may be in the category of those who are prone to develop problems with addictive substances.
		If pain medications are determined to be indicated, it is generally helpful to provide these on a scheduled basis rather than on an as-needed basis, since this latter approach may reinforce pain preoccupation.
		It is recommended that consideration be given to the prescription of an antidepressant medication to treat @'s pain and depressive symptoms. Research indicates that antidepressants may directly improve tolerance for pain apart from any effect on depression. In addition, by reducing depression, such medication may improve @'s ability to cope with pain. If an antidepressant with strong sedative properties is prescribed, this may also contribute to a reduction in sleep disturbance (i.e., early morning awakening or difficulty falling asleep due to pain).

(continued)

Section	Topic	Text
		@'s medical doctors may wish to consider use of antidepressant medication for relief of pain and associated sleep disturbance.
	Psychotropic Medication	
		@ should be referred to a psychiatrist for further psychopharmacological treatment, including possible combination and augmentation strategies.
		I recommend evaluation and treatment by a psychiatrist experienced in working with persons who have sustained neurological injury.
		Psychiatric consultation is recommended to evaluate the feasibility of psychopharmacological interventions for @'s symptoms.
		As @ has evidently obtained prescriptions from multiple providers, it is recommended that a careful review be done of current medications to ensure that side effects of drug interactions are not adversely affecting cognition.
		It is possible that @'s medications (e.g., ***) may be interfering with cognitive functioning. @ did report that the development of cognitive problems has roughly coincided with the use of these medications. If this is in fact the case, it may be helpful for medical providers to re-evaluate @'s medication needs. @ has been advised to discuss this issue with medical providers but has been cautioned not to make any change in medication except under a physician's advice.
		Given @'s reports of sleep disturbance and memory problems, a moderately sedating antidepressant with minimal anticholinergic side effects may be helpful.
		The continued presence of dysphoric mood and other signs of depression (i.e., ***) suggest, that antidepressant medication be considered for @.
		Extra attention may need to be given to educating @ about the importance of taking antidepressant medication regularly as prescribed and for a sufficient period of time to establish its efficiency.
		Given previous apparently unsuccessful attempts at antidepressant treatment, a thorough medication history would be useful. Detailed knowledge about dosages of previous antidepressants, the duration of trials with these medications, and any troublesome side effects would be helpful in selecting an appropriate antidepressant for @.

(continued)

Section	Topic	Text
	Psychotherapy	
		Individuals with similar levels of emotional distress often benefit from psychotherapy.
		Because of the long commute to ***, it would be helpful to try to find a more local treatment provider, and I recommend contacting ***.
		The treatment sessions recommended by Dr. *** are appropriate and will be scheduled.
		Psychotherapy is recommended to treat depression and assist in the resolution of grief over the numerous losses @ has experienced.
		To be maximally effective, treatment should also involve @'s family.
		@ will require supportive, problem-focused psychotherapy that takes into account the presence of memory, attention, and processing limitations. Treatment should be obtained, if possible, from a neuropsychologist, clinical psychologist or other psychotherapist familiar with the emotional, social, cognitive, and behavioral sequelae of brain injury.
		@ does not require intensive psychotherapy. However, I would recommend less frequent sessions with a neuropsychologist, clinical psychologist, or other psychotherapist familiar with the issues that surround brain injury such as frustration tolerance, anger management, deficit awareness, and self-esteem.
		There does not appear to be a need for psychological intervention at this time, but @'s adjustment status should be periodically monitored by physicians, as lessening of denial over time may be accompanied by increased dysphoria. If this occurs, referral back to a mental health provider is recommended.
		Over time, with increased awareness of deficits and their implications, @ may become more depressed, and it would be helpful for supportive counseling to be available at that time.
		@'s level of distress is high enough to warrant referral for individual psychotherapy. Treatment sessions are usually provided on a one-hour-per-week basis, and I expect @ to need approximately *** sessions.
		Practitioners skilled at this type of treatment include: ***.

Appendix: Glasscow Comma Scale Scoring Key

Instructions for scoring:

Compare your responses to those suggested below. Assign 1 point for each knowledge (K), writing ability (W), and common sense (C) correction and 6 points for each follow-through (F) task completed, for a maximum score of 80.

Wudzit Taique, a 47 year old Latvian woman recently provisionally

W	Compound adjectives that precede the word they modify are hyphenated: 47-year-old Latvian	

diagnosed with Dementia of the Alzheimer's Type (DAT) was referred by

K	Diagnoses and diseases are not routinely capitalized except when acronyms or people's names: dementia of the Alzheimer's type (DAT)	
W	Parenthetical phrases are set off by commas: Wudzit Taique, a ....(DAT), was referred	

Dr. Edward S. Hands, M.D. for this 01/01/2011 neuropychological evaluation.

W	It is redundant to use both "Dr." and "M.D.": Edward S. Hands, M.D.	
W	Academic degrees are set off by commas: Hands, M.D., for …	
K	Spell correctly: neuropsychological tvian	

Prior to her symptom onset, Ms. Taique reported being extremely active (i.e.

C	We do not know what she reported before the onset: Ms. Taique reported that prior to her dementia	
W	Use "i.e." when the list is exhaustive, which this list clearly is not. When listing examples, use "e.g."	
W	Both abbreviations are typically followed by commas: e.g.,	

R.L. Wanlass, *The Neuropsychology Toolkit: Guidelines, Formats, and Language*, DOI 10.1007/ 978-1-4614-1882-5, © Springer Science+Business Media, LLC 2012

liked to paint, make stained glass, and attending the opera) but she tearfully

W	Items in a series should be of parallel grammatical form: paint, make …, and attend	
W	Compound sentences normally require a comma before the conjunction that joins them: opera), but	
K	Point out potential exposure to neurotoxins (e.g., lead used in making stained glass)	

related that she is no longer interested in these hobbies. Her recent activities have consisted only of sipping vodka and watching Fox News.

K	Point out possible contribution of vodka to impaired cognition and/or mood issues	
C	Attribute to a source such implausible statements ("only" activities) so you do not appear gullible	

Her husband, a long-haul tractor-trailer driver and stamp collector, reports

C	Point out potential safety concern for patient with husband being away long periods driving a truck	
C	Eliminate irrelevant information such as "stamp collector"	
W	His reporting is presumably not an ongoing activity or state: use "reported" not "reports"	

observing cognitive symptoms in his wife for the past six months. He also said

K	Symptoms are reported; signs are observed	
C	Reference to "cognitive symptoms" is too vague; examples are needed	

she will emit gasping and snorting sounds when she sleeps.

W	Future tense is not needed: she emits	
K	Need to rule out sleep apnea with possible hypoxia should be noted	

They live locally with there preschool-age grandchild, who they adopted

W	Use correct possessive form: their	
C	Indicate recognition of potential safety concerns for young child in this environment	
W	Use "whom" because the grandchild is not the one who did the adopting	

following the death of the child's parents last year.

C	Point out possible role of grief over loss of child as causal factor for Ms. Taique's behavior change	

Ms. Taique immigrated from Latvia two years ago. She completed 12 years

W	When someone leaves a country, it is considered "emigration" from that country	

of schooling in Russian and Mining Technology. She then worked as a coal minor

W	Fields of study or work are not typically capitalized, except for languages: Russian and mining …	
W	Spell correctly: miner	

for several years until developing chronic back pain from a 1975 mining accident.

C	This date indicates that she was implausibly young when working in a mine	
C	Indicate whether accident caused cognitive or psychological sequelae (e.g., head injury or PTSD)	

Currently prescribed medications consist of Oxycontin, Nardil, and

K	Potential interactions involving alcohol and these medications should be noted	
K	Potential contribution of medications to altered cognition and behavior should be noted	
K	OxyContin has two capital letters	

Hydrocodone, and she discontinued Luvox two days ago due to side affects.

K	Generic drug names are not generally capitalized: hydrocodone	
K	Danger of interaction between SSRI and MAO inhibiter should be noted	
W	Do not confuse affects with effects	

She also takes about two asprin every four to six hours.

K	Spell correctly: aspirin	

Ms. Taique's vision was determined to be adequate to participate in testing, as was her hearing, despite her complaint of tinnitis. Test results are considered

K	Point out potential contribution of aspirin to tinnitus	
K	Spell correctly: tinnitus	

a valid reflection of her current cognitive ability.

K	Effort testing is generally considered important before reaching this conclusion about test validity	
C	Linguistic and cultural confounds need to be considered	

| C | Address possible influence of medications, alcohol consumption, and pain on test results | |

Her Full Scale IQ is 112 (VCI = 107; PRI = 103; WMI = 104; PSI = 105).

| C | The Full Scale IQ could not be that high given these index scores | |

Thus, Ms. Taique's current overall intellectual functioning tested as superior, with

| K | A score of 112 is not generally regarded as superior | |

verbal abilities significantly stronger than nonverbal abilities. She demonstrated

| K | This difference between Verbal Comprehension and Perceptual Reasoning scores is not statistically significant | |

relative strength in arithmetic, as indicated by her Digit Span scaled score of 12,

| K | Arithmetic ability is not measured by Digit Span | |
| K | A scaled score of 12 would not indicate a relative strength given the IQ scores listed above | |

which falls at the 84th%ile. On the Trail Making Test, Mr. Taique scored in the

K	The 84th%ile corresponds to a scaled score of 13, not 12	
K	Specify Trails A or Trails B	
W	Ms. not Mr.	

mild-deficit range (32nd%ile) compared to others her age group, however, this

C	The 32nd%ile would generally be considered in the normal range	
W	...compared to others in her age group...	
W	"However" is not a conjunction; use "but" or place a semi-colon before "however"	

measure is not particularly sensitive to neurologic dysfunction. Language abilities

| K | This test generally is considered sensitive to neurologic dysfunction | |

appeared intact, as performance on multiple measures of reading, spelling, comprehension, design fluency, and word-finding abilities were normal. Memory

| K | Design fluency is not generally considered a measure of language ability | |
| W | Performance was normal; subject and verb must agree | |

testing revealed deficits in list learning and free recall, while recognition tested as normal, suggesting problems involving both retention and retrieval.

K	If free recall is poor but recognition is normal, this suggests retrieval but not retention problems	

Ms. Taique scored in the normal range (T=67) on Scale 7 of the MMPI-2,

W	MMPI-2 T-scores of 67 are not generally considered normal	

and there are no other indications of depression.

K	Scale 7 is not considered primarily a measure of depression	
C	Reference to "no other indications of depression" contradicts previous statement about tearfulness	
C	This conclusion also contradicts previous statement about loss if interest in hobbies	

In conclusion, assessment results are consistent with a diagnosis of DAT.

C	This conclusion ignores other possible causal factors	

F	Wrote name	
F	Wrote date	
F	Switched ink	

Index

CPSIA information can be obtained at www.ICGtesting.com
Printed in the USA
LVOW07*1138271015

459944LV00011B/315/P